LECTURE NOTES ON

Dermatology

ROBIN GRAHAM-BROWN

BSc, MB, BS (Lond), FRCP
Consultant Dermatologist,
The Leicester Royal Infirmary, Leicester,
and Honorary Senior Lecturer in Dermatology,
University of Leicester School of Medicine

TONY BURNS

MB, BS (Lond), FRCP
Consultant Dermatologist,
The Leicester Royal Infirmary, Leicester,
and Honorary Senior Lecturer in Dermatology,
University of Leicester School of Medicine

Seventh edition

b

**Blackwell
Science**

To all medical students, and to our children:
James, Matthew, John Joseph and David.

© 1965, 1969, 1973, 1977, 1983, 1990, 1996 by
Blackwell Science Ltd
Editorial Offices:
Osney Mead, Oxford OX2 0EL
25 John Street, London WC1N 2BL
23 Ainslie Place, Edinburgh EH3 6AJ
238 Main Street, Cambridge
 Massachusetts 02142, USA
54 University Street, Carlton
 Victoria 3053, Australia

Other Editorial Offices:
Arnette Blackwell SA
 224, Boulevard Saint Germain
 75007 Paris, France

Blackwell Wissenschafts-Verlag GmbH
 Kurfürstendamm 57
 10707 Berlin, Germany

 Zehetnergasse 6
 A-1140 Wien
 Austria

First published 1965
Second edition 1969
Third edition 1973
Fourth edition 1977
Fifth edition 1983
Sixth edition 1990
Seventh edition 1996

Set by Excel Typesetters Co., Hong Kong
Printed and bound in Italy by
G. Canale & C. S.p.A., Turin

The Blackwell Science logo
is a trade mark of
Blackwell Science Ltd,
registered at the
United Kingdom Trade
Marks Registry

DISTRIBUTORS
 Marston Book Services Ltd
 PO Box 269
 Abingdon
 Oxon OX14 4YN
 (Orders: Tel: 01235 465500
   Fax: 01235 465555)

USA
 Blackwell Science, Inc.
 238 Main Street
 Cambridge, MA 02142
 (Orders: Tel: 800 215-1000
    617 876-7000
   Fax: 617 492-5263)

Canada
 Copp Clark, Ltd
 2775 Matheson Blvd East
 Mississauga, Ontario
 Canada, L4W 4P7
 (Orders: Tel: 800 263-4374
    905 238-6074)

Australia
 Blackwell Science Pty Ltd
 54 University Street
 Carlton, Victoria 3053
 (Orders: Tel: 03 9347 0300
   Fax: 03 9349 3016)

A catalogue record for this title
is available from the British Library

ISBN 0-86542-635-X (BSL)
 0-86542-709-7 (IE)

Library of Congress
Cataloging-in-publication Data

Graham-Brown, R.A.C. (Robin A.C.)
 Lecture notes on dermatology.—7th ed./
 Robin Graham-Brown, Tony Burns.
  p. cm.
 Rev. ed. of: Lectures notes on dermatology/
 Bethel Solomons. 5th ed. 1983.
 Includes bibliographical references and index.
 ISBN 0-86542-635-X.—ISBN 0-86542-635-X
 1. Dermatology—Outlines, syllabi, etc.
 2. Skin—Diseases—Outlines, syllabi, etc.
 I. Graham-Brown, R.A.C. (Robin A.C.)
 II. Burns, Tony, FRCP. III. Solomons, Bethel.
 Lecture notes on dermatology. IV. Title.
 [DNLM: 1. Skin Diseases.
 WR 140 G742L 1996]
 RL74.3.G73 1996
 616.5—dc20
 DNLM/DLC
 for Library of Congress   95-51162
                CIP

Contents

Preface

In this, the seventh edition of *Lecture Notes on Dermatology*, we have modified the format of the previous edition to some extent, in order to highlight key parts of the text. We have, however, endeavoured to preserve the concept of 'user-friendly' readability which was one of our primary aims with the sixth edition. The sections concerning therapy have been updated to include recent advances in treatment.

We hope that this text will be of value not only to medical students, but also to general practitioners, and nurses involved in the care of dermatology patients. We also hope that exposure to *Lecture Notes on Dermatology*, together with clinical contact with patients suffering from skin disease, will prompt a deeper interest in this important medical specialty.

Robin Graham-Brown
Tony Burns

Acknowledgements

We would like to thank Drs Imrich Sarkany and Charles Calnan, under whose guidance we both learned dermatology, and are grateful to them for some of the illustrations. We are also grateful to our students, who remind us constantly of the importance of clarity in communication. Finally, we thank Peter Saugman, who offered us the opportunity to write this book, and all the staff at Blackwell Science who have helped us patiently through the editing and production stages.

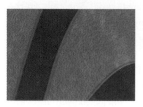

CHAPTER I

Structure and Function of the Skin, Hair and Nails

Skin, skin is a wonderful thing,
Keeps the outside out and the inside in.

It is essential to have some background knowledge of the normal structure and function of any organ before you can hope to understand the abnormal. Skin is the icing on the anatomical cake, and without it not only would we all look rather unappealing, but a variety of unpleasant physiological phenomena would bring about our demise. Hopefully, by the end of this first chapter you will have been persuaded that the skin is quite a remarkable organ, and that you are lucky to be on such intimate terms with it.

SKIN STRUCTURE

The skin is composed of two layers, the epidermis and the dermis. The epidermis, which is the outer layer, and its appendages (hair, nails, sebaceous glands and sweat glands), are derived from the embryonic ectoderm. The dermis is of mesodermal origin.

The epidermis

The epidermis is a multilayered structure which renews itself continuously by cell division in its deepest layer—the basal layer. The principal cell type is the epidermal cell, commonly referred to as a 'keratinocyte'. The cells produced by cell division in the basal layer constitute the prickle cell layer and, as they ascend towards the surface, they synthesize the fibrous protein keratin. A cell takes approximately 30 days to pass from the basal layer to the surface of the epidermis (epidermal transit time). The cells on the surface of the skin, which constitute the horny layer (stratum corneum), are keratinized dead cells which are gradually abraded by daily wear and tear.

Look at the layers more closely (Fig. 1.1). The basal layer is composed of columnar cells which are anchored to a basement membrane. This is a multilayered structure from which anchoring fibrils extend into the superficial dermis. Interspersed amongst the basal cells are melanocytes—large dendritic cells derived from the neural crest—which are responsible for melanin pigment production. Melanocytes contain cytoplasmic organelles called melanosomes, in which melanin is synthesized from tyrosine. The melanosomes migrate along the dendrites, and are transferred to the keratinocytes in the prickle cell layer. In white people the melanosomes are grouped together in 'melanosome complexes', and they gradually degenerate as the keratinocytes move towards the surface of the skin. In black people, the skin contains the same number of melanocytes as that of white people, but the melanosomes are larger, remain separate, and persist throughout the full thickness of the epidermis. The main stimulus to melanin production is ultraviolet (UV) radiation.

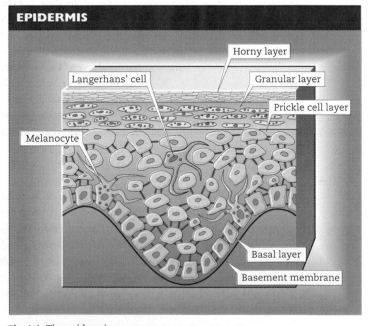

Fig. 1.1 The epidermis.

Melanin protects the cell nuclei in the epidermis from the harmful effects of UV radiation. A sun tan is a natural protective mechanism, not a cosmetic boon! Skin cancer is extremely uncommon in dark-skinned races, because their skin is protected from UV damage by large quantities of melanin. This is not the case in the pale, pimply, lager-swilling advert for British manhood who dashes onto the beach in Majorca and flash-fries himself to lobster thermidor on day 1 of his annual holiday.

The prickle cell layer acquires its name from the spiky appearance produced by intercellular bridges (desmosomes) which connect adjacent cells. Scattered throughout the prickle cell layer are Langerhans' cells. These dendritic cells are probably modified macrophages which originate in the bone marrow and migrate to the epidermis. They are the first line of immunological defence against environmental antigens, and are responsible for the uptake of such antigens and their presentation to immunocompetent lymphocytes so that an immune response can be mounted.

Above the prickle cell layer is the granular layer, which is composed of flattened cells containing numerous darkly staining particles known as keratohyalin granules. Also present in the cytoplasm of cells in the granular layer are organelles known as lamellar granules (Odland bodies). These contain lipids and enzymes, and they discharge their contents into the intercellular spaces between the cells of the granular layer and stratum corneum—providing the equivalent of 'mortar' between the cellular 'bricks'.

The cells of the stratum corneum are flattened, keratinized cells which are devoid of nuclei and cytoplasmic organelles. Adjacent cells overlap at their margins, and this locking together of cells, together with intercellular lipid, forms a very effective barrier. The stratum corneum varies in thickness according to the region of the body. It is thickest on the palms of the hands and soles of the feet.

KERATIN PRODUCTION

Keratin is the main epidermal structural protein. Keratinocytes in the basal and prickle cell layers synthesize keratin filaments (tonofilaments) which aggregate into bundles (tonofibrils). Eventually, in the cells of the stratum corneum, these bundles of keratin filaments form a complex intracellular network embedded in an amorphous protein matrix which is derived from the keratohyalin granules of the granular layer. The keratinized epidermis forms a barrier which is relatively impermeable to substances passing in or out of the body.

EPIDERMAL APPENDAGES

The eccrine and apocrine sweat glands, the hair and sebaceous glands, and the nails, constitute the epidermal appendages.

Eccrine sweat glands

Eccrine sweat glands are important in body temperature regulation. A human has from 2 to 3 million eccrine sweat glands covering almost all the body surface. They are particularly numerous on the palms of the hands and soles of the feet. Each consists of a secretory coil deep in the dermis, and a duct which conveys the sweat to the surface. Eccrine glands secrete water, electrolytes, lactate, urea and ammonia. The secretory coil produces isotonic sweat, but sodium chloride is reabsorbed in the duct so that sweat reaching the surface is hypotonic. Patients suffering from cystic fibrosis have defective resorption of sodium chloride, and rapidly become salt-depleted in a hot environment. Eccrine sweat glands are innervated by the sympathetic nervous system, but the neurotransmitter is acetylcholine.

Apocrine sweat glands

Apocrine sweat glands are found principally in the axillae and anogenital region. Specialized apocrine glands include the wax glands of the ear and the milk glands of the breast. Apocrine glands are also composed of a secretory coil and a duct, but the duct opens into a hair follicle, not directly onto the surface of the skin. Apocrine glands produce an oily secretion containing protein, carbohydrate, ammonia and lipid. These glands become active at puberty, and secretion is controlled by adrenergic nerve fibres. Pungent axillary body odour (axillary bromhidrosis) is the result of the action of bacteria on apocrine secretions. In some animals apocrine secretions are important sexual attractants, but the average human armpit provides a different type of overwhelming olfactory experience.

Hair

Hairs grow out of tubular invaginations of the epidermis known as follicles, and a hair follicle and its associated sebaceous glands are referred to as a 'pilosebaceous unit'. There are three types of hair: lanugo hair is present *in utero* and is shed by the 8th month of fetal life; vellus hair is the fine downy hair which covers most of the body except those areas occupied by terminal hair; terminal hair is the thick pigmented hair of the scalp, beard, eyebrows, eyelashes, axillae and pubic area. In some areas, such as the beard, axillae and pubic region, the development of terminal hair is under hormonal control—the hairs in these areas are vellus until the onset of puberty. On the scalp, the reverse occurs in male pattern balding—terminal hair becomes vellus hair. In men, terminal hair on the body usually increases in amount as middle-age strikes, and hairy ears are a puzzling accompaniment of advancing years—it is difficult to imagine what biological advantage this might confer.

Hair follicles extend into the dermis at an angle (Fig. 1.2). A small bundle of smooth muscle fibres, the arrector pili muscle, extends from just beneath the epidermis and is attached to the side of the follicle at an angle. Arrector pili muscles are supplied by adrenergic nerves, and are responsible for the erection of hairs during cold or emotional stress ('goose flesh'; horripilation). The duct of the sebaceous gland enters the follicle just above the point of attachment of the arrector pili muscle. At the lower end of the follicle is the hair bulb, part of which, the hair matrix, is a zone of rapidly dividing cells which is responsible for the formation of the hair shaft. Hair pigment is produced by melanocytes in the hair bulb. Cells produced in the hair bulb become densely packed, elongated and arranged parallel to the long axis of the hair shaft. They gradually become keratinized as they ascend in the hair follicle. The main part of each hair fibre is the cortex, which is composed of keratinized spindle-shaped cells (Fig. 1.3). Terminal hairs have a central core known as the medulla, consisting of

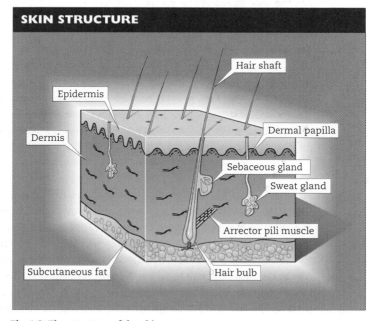

Fig. 1.2 The structure of the skin.

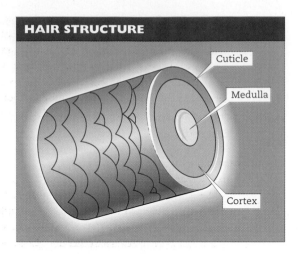

HAIR STRUCTURE

Cuticle

Medulla

Cortex

Fig. 1.3 The structure of hair.

specialized cells which contain air spaces. Covering the cortex is the cuticle, a thin layer of cells which overlap like the tiles on a roof, with the free margins of the cells pointing towards the tip of the hair. The cross-sectional shape of hair varies with body site and with race. Negroid hair is distinctly oval in cross-section, and pubic, beard and eyelash hairs have an oval cross-section in all racial types.

The growth of each hair is cyclical—periods of active growth alternate with resting phases. After each period of active growth (anagen) there is a short resting phase (telogen), following which the follicle reactivates, a new hair is produced, and the old hair is shed. The duration of these cyclical phases depends on the age of the individual and the location of the follicle on the body. The duration of anagen in a scalp follicle is genetically determined, and ranges from 2 to >5 years. This is why some women can grow very long hair, whereas others cannot. Scalp hair telogen lasts from 3 to 4 months. The daily growth rate of scalp hair is approximately 0.35 mm. The activity of each follicle is independent of that of its neighbours. At any one time approximately 85% of scalp hairs are in anagen, and 15% in telogen. The average number of hairs shed daily is 100. In areas other than the scalp anagen is relatively short—if this was not the case we should all be kept busy clipping eyebrows, eyelashes and nether regions.

Shaving does not increase the hair growth rate or encourage 'thicker' hair, nor does hair continue growing after death—shrinkage of soft tissues around the hair produces this illusion.

Human hair colour is produced by two types of melanin—eumelanins in black and brown hair, and phaeomelanins in auburn and blond hair.

Greying of hair is the result of a gradual decrease in tyrosinase activity in the melanocytes of the hair bulb. The age of onset of greying is genetically determined, but other factors may be involved such as auto-immunity—premature greying of the hair is a recognized association of pernicious anaemia. The phenomenon of 'going white overnight', usually attributed to a severe fright, is physically impossible. It would, however, be feasible to 'go white' over a period of a few days by selective loss of pigmented hairs.

Sebaceous glands

Sebaceous glands are found everywhere on the skin apart from the hands and feet. They are particularly numerous and prominent on the head and neck, the chest, and the back. Sebaceous glands are part of the pilosebaceous unit, and their lipid-rich secretion (sebum) flows through a duct into the hair follicle. Modified sebaceous glands which open directly on the surface are found on the eyelids, lips, nipples, glans penis and prepuce, and the buccal mucosa (Fordyce spots). They are holocrine glands—sebum is produced by disintegration of glandular cells rather than an active secretory process.

Sebaceous glands are prominent at birth, under the influence of maternal hormones, but atrophy soon after, and do not enlarge again until puberty. Enlargement of the glands and sebum production at puberty are stimulated by androgens. Growth hormone and thyroid hormones also affect sebum production.

Nails

A nail is a transparent plate of keratin derived from an invagination of epidermis on the dorsum of the terminal phalanx of a digit (Fig. 1.4). The nail plate is the product of cell division in the nail matrix, which lies deep to the proximal nail fold, but is partly visible as the pale 'half moon' (lunula) at the base of the nail. The nail plate is firmly adherent to the underlying nail bed. The cuticle is an extension of the horny layer of the proximal nail fold onto the nail plate. It forms a seal between the nail plate and proximal nail fold, preventing penetration of extraneous material.

Nail growth is continuous throughout life, but is more rapid in youth than in old age. The average rate of growth of fingernails is approximately 1 mm per week, and the time taken for a finger nail to grow from matrix to free edge is about 6 months. Nails on the dominant hand grow slightly more rapidly than those on the non-dominant hand. Toenails grow at about one-third the rate of fingernails, and take 18 months to grow from matrix to free edge.

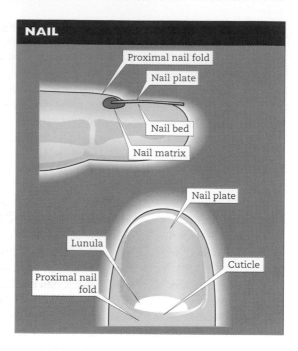

Fig. 1.4 The nail.

Many factors affect nail growth rate. It is increased in psoriasis, and may be speeded up in the presence of inflammatory change around the nail. A severe systemic upset can produce a sudden slowing of nail growth, and growth may be considerably slowed in a hand immobilized in plaster.

The dermis

The dermis is a layer of connective tissue lying beneath the epidermis, and forms the bulk of the skin. The dermis and epidermis interdigitate via downward epidermal projections (rete ridges), and upward dermal projections (dermal papillae) (Fig. 1.2). The main feature of the dermis is a network of interlacing fibres, mostly collagen, but with some elastin. These fibres give the dermis great strength and elasticity. The collagen and elastin fibres, which are protein, are embedded in a ground substance of mucopolysaccharides (glycosaminoglycans).

The main cells are fibroblasts, mast cells, and macrophages. Fibroblasts synthesize the connective tissue matrix of the dermis, and are usually found in close proximity to collagen and elastin fibres. Mast cells are specialized secretory cells present throughout the dermis, but they are more numerous around blood vessels and appendages. They contain granules whose contents include mediators such as histamine, prostaglandins, leukotrienes and eosinophil and neutrophil chemotactic factors. Macrophages are phagocytic cells which originate in the bone marrow, and they act as scavengers of cell debris and extracellular material.

The dermis is also richly supplied with blood vessels, lymphatics, nerves, and sensory receptors.

Beneath the dermis, a layer of subcutaneous fat separates the skin from underlying fascia and muscle.

DERMATOGLYPHICS

Fingerprints, the characteristic elevated ridge patterns on the fingertips of humans, are unique to each individual. The fingers and toes, and the palms and soles, are covered with a system of ridges which form patterns. The term 'dermatoglyphics' is applied to the configurations of the ridges. If you look closely at your hands you will see these tiny ridges, which are separate from the skin creases. On the tips of the fingers there are three basic patterns: arches, loops and whorls (Fig. 1.5). The loops are sub-divided into ulnar or radial, depending on whether the loop is open to the ulnar or radial side of the hand. A triangular intersection of these ridges is known as a triradius, and these triradii are not only present on finger-tips, but also at the base of each finger, and usually on the proximal part of the palm.

Not only are the ridge patterns of fingerprints useful for the identification of criminals, but characteristic dermatoglyphic abnormalities frequently accompany many chromosomal aberrations.

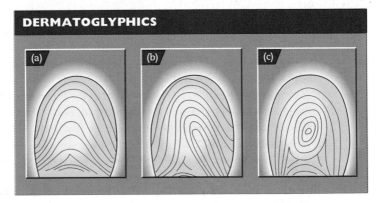

DERMATOGLYPHICS

(a)   (b)   (c)

Fig. 1.5 Dermatoglyphics: (a) arch; (b) loop; (c) whorl.

FUNCTIONS OF THE SKIN

Skin is like wax paper that holds everything in without dripping. (Art Linkletter, *A Child's Garden of Misinformation*, 1965)

It is obvious from the complex structure of the skin that it is not there simply to hold all the other bits together. Some of the functions of skin are listed as follows:

SKIN FUNCTIONS

- Prevents loss of essential body fluids
- Protects against entry of toxic environmental chemicals and microorganisms
- Protects against damage from UV radiation
- Regulates body temperature
- Synthesis of vitamin D
- Important in sexual attraction and social interaction

In the absence of a stratum corneum we would lose significant amounts of water to the environment, and rapidly become dehydrated. If the stratum corneum is removed by stripping with tape, water loss to the environment increases 10-fold or more.

The stratum corneum is also quite an effective barrier to the penetration of external agents. However, this barrier capacity is considerably reduced if the stratum corneum is hydrated, or its lipid content is reduced by the use of lipid solvents. The structural integrity of the stratum corneum also protects against invasion by microorganisms.

The protective effect of melanin against UV damage has already been mentioned.

The skin is a vital part of the body's temperature regulation system. The body's core temperature is regulated by the hypothalamus. The response of the skin to cold is vasoconstriction and a marked reduction in blood flow, decreasing transfer of heat to the body surface. The response to heat is vasodilation, an increase in skin blood flow, and loss of heat to the environment. Perspiration helps to cool the body by evaporation of sweat. These thermoregulatory functions of the skin are impaired in certain skin diseases—patients suffering from exfoliative dermatitis radiate heat to their environment because their skin blood flow is considerably increased—and they are unable to control this by vasoconstriction. In a cold environment their central core temperature drops and they may die of hypothermia.

The skin is also a huge sensory receptor, perceiving heat, cold, pain, temperature, light touch, and pressure.

Vitamin D (cholecalciferol) is produced in the skin by the action of UV light on dehydrocholesterol. In those whose diets are deficient in vitamin D this extra source of the vitamin can be important.

In addition to all these mechanistic functions, the skin plays an essential aesthetic role in social interaction and sexual attraction.

Hence, you can see that your skin is doing a good job. Apart from looking pleasant, it is saving you from becoming a cold, UV-damaged, brittle-boned, desiccated prune.

CHAPTER 2

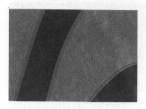

Approach to the Diagnosis of Dermatological Disease

Baglivi has said, 'The patient is the doctor's best text-book'. That 'text-book' however has to be introduced to the student and those who effect the introductions are not always wise. (Dannie Abse, Doctors and Patients)
The dermatologist's art is giving a disease a long Greek name . . . and then a topical steroid. (Anon)

INTRODUCTION

Dermatology is essentially a clinical specialty, and it is important for any aspiring clinician to realize that, in order to be able to prescribe treatment and/or offer any useful prognostic information about a patient's problem, he or she must first make a diagnosis. This chapter is about that process in relation to dermatological disorders.

THE VALUE OF A DIAGNOSIS

The facts on which a clinician makes his or her diagnosis *must* always come first and foremost from the patient and there is, therefore, no substitute for talking to and examining patients. This is especially true of skin disease.

A diagnosis is a short statement about a disease state or condition.

DIAGNOSIS

- Provides a working label which will be recognized by others
- Implies some commonality with other patients with the same disease state or condition. This may be in aetiology, histopathology, clinical features or in responsiveness to treatment
- Offers a prognosis and information about contagion or heredity
- Gives access to treatment modalities

DERMATOLOGICAL DIAGNOSIS

That which we call a rose,
by any other name would smell as sweet.
    (Shakespeare, *Romeo and Juliet*)

Aspiring dermatologists must begin by becoming familiar with the diagnostic labels used in the description and classification of skin disease. This can seem daunting at first glance but remember that currently accepted diagnostic entities in medicine are all bound by convention. Dermatology is no different from other specialties, except perhaps in the degree to which subtle clinical variations are afforded separate names. Names given to disease have emerged by general consensus from hundreds of years of attempts at classification and categorization. The fact that diagnostic terms often bear no relationship to modern thinking is not of itself important. An apple is still an apple, even if we don't know who first called it that or why!

Therefore, as in any other branch of medicine, the diagnostic terminology in use in dermatology has to be learned. This is not as hard as it may at first seem. In the same way as a visitor to Mars will have to become familiar with what things on Mars are called, so an aspiring dermatologist will rapidly become acquainted with commoner skin diseases (e.g. eczema, psoriasis or warts). In time, he or she will also begin to recognize rarer disorders and less 'classical' variants of the commoner ones. However, this remains a dynamic process which involves seeing, reading, asking and learning—always with the eyes, ears and mind open!

The steps to making a dermatological diagnosis

In principle there is nothing difficult about dermatological diagnosis. As with any other specialty, the process of identifying skin diseases consists of taking a history, examining the patient, and performing investigations where necessary. In practice many dermatologists will ask questions *after* a quick look to assess the problem, and also during the formal examination. However, we should consider the elements of the process separately.

A dermatological history contains most of the questions which you are used to asking, such as onset and duration, fluctuation, nature of symptoms, past history, etc. There are some differences, however, which are largely in the emphasis placed on certain aspects, shown as follows:

DERMATOLOGICAL HISTORY

Past history
Include general problems, such as
- Diabetes and TB
- Past skin problems
- Significant allergies

Family history
- Some disorders are infectious; others have strong genetic backgrounds

Occupation and hobbies
- The skin is frequently affected by materials encountered at work and in the home

Therapy
- Not only *systemic* medication but also *topical*; many patients apply multiple creams and ointments; topicals may be medicinal (patients nearly always forget their names)
BUT
- Topicals may also be self-chosen as part of a 'cosmetic' regimen

There are also specific features of dermatological histories which you should watch out for.

SYMPTOMS

Patients with skin disease talk about symptoms, such as itching, which you may not have met before. You will have to learn to assess and quantify these. You will soon get used to this. For example, a severe itch will keep patients awake or stop them from concentrating at work.

PATIENTS' LANGUAGE

Be careful about terms which patients use to describe their skin problems. In our part of England weals are often called 'blisters' and it is easy to be misled. Always ask the patient to describe precisely what he or she means by a specific term.

QUALITY OF LIFE

It may be helpful to assess the impact of the problem on the patient's normal daily activities and self-image: work, school, sleep, self-confidence, personal relationships.

PATIENT PRECONCEPTIONS

Patients often have their own ideas about the cause of skin problems and will readily offer them! For example, washing powder is almost universally considered to be a major cause of rashes, and injuries to be triggers of skin tumours. You will have to sieve such information in the light of your findings.

Watch out, too, for the very high expectations of many patients. They know that visible evidence is there for all to see: dermatology often truly requires a 'spot' diagnosis! Everyone from the patient and his/her relatives to the local greengrocer or policeman can see the problem and express their opinion.

EXAMINATION

The next step is to examine the patient. Wise counsels maintain that you should *always* examine a patient from head to foot. In reality this can be hard on both patient and doctor, especially if the presenting complaint is a solitary wart on the thumb! However, as a general rule, and especially with inflammatory dermatoses and conditions where there are several lesions, it is important to have an overall look at the sites involved. You may also encounter unexpected findings, such as melanomas and other skin cancers.

Inspect *and palpate* the lesion(s) or rash (it may help to use a magnifying hand lens). The fundamental elements of a good dermatological examination are:

1 site and/or distribution of the problem;
2 characteristics of individual lesion(s);
3 examination of 'secondary' sites;
4 'special' techniques.

DERMATOLOGICAL ASSESSMENT

1 Site(s) and/or distribution
This can be very helpful: for example, psoriasis has a predilection for knees, elbows, scalp and lower back; eczema favours the flexures in children; acne occurs predominantly on the face and upper trunk; basal cell carcinomata are more common on the head and neck

2 Characteristics of individual lesion(s)
The type
Some simple preliminary reading is essential. Use Table 2.1 for the most common and important terms and their definitions

The size, shape, outline and border
Size is best *measured*, rather than being compared to peas, oranges or coins of the realm
Lesions may be various shapes, e.g. round, oval, annular, linear or 'irregular'; straight edges and angles may suggest external factors
The border is well defined in psoriasis, but blurred in most patches of eczema

The colour
It is always useful to note the colour: red, purple, brown, slate-black, etc.

Surface features (Table 2.1)
It is helpful to assess whether the surface is smooth or rough, and to distinguish crust (dried serum) from scale (hyperkeratosis); some assessment of scale can be helpful, e.g. 'silvery' in psoriasis

The texture—superficial? deep?
Use your fingertips on the surface; assess the depth and position in or beneath the skin; lift scale or crust to see what is underneath; try to make the lesion blanch with pressure

3 Secondary sites
Look for additional features which may assist in diagnosis. Good examples of this include:
- the nails in psoriasis
- the fingers and wrists in scabies
- the toe-webs in fungal infections
- the mouth in lichen planus

4 'Special' techniques
These will be covered in the appropriate chapters, but there are some tricks, e.g.:
- scraping a psoriatic plaque for capillary bleeding
- the Nikolsky sign in blistering diseases
- 'diascopy' in suspected cutaneous tuberculosis

LESION CHARACTERISTICS

Types of lesion
- Macule: a flat, circumscribed area of skin discolouration
- Papule: a circumscribed elevation of the skin less than 0.5 cm in diameter
- Nodule: a circumscribed visible or palpable lump, larger than 0.5 cm
- Plaque: a circumscribed, disc-shaped, elevated area of skin:
  'small' <2 cm in diameter
  'large' >2 cm in diameter
- Vesicle: a small visible collection of fluid (less than 0.5 cm in diameter)
- Bulla: a large visible collection of fluid (over 0.5 cm)
- Pustule: a visible accumulation of pus
- Ulcer: a loss of epidermis (often with loss of underlying dermis and subcutis as well)
- Weal: a circumscribed, elevated area of cutaneous oedema

Surface characteristics
- Scale: visible and palpable flakes due to aggregation and/or abnormalities of shed epidermal cells
- Crust: accumulated dried exudate, e.g. serum
- Horn: an elevated projection of keratin
- Excoriation: a secondary, superficial ulceration, due to scratching
- Maceration: an appearance of surface softening due to constant wetting
- Lichenification: a flat-topped thickening of the skin often secondary to scratching

Table 2.1 Types and characteristics of lesions.

Unfortunately, names and terms appear to get in the way of learning in dermatology more than in some specialties. Indeed this seems to be one reason why many clinicians claim that dermatology is a mysterious and impenetrable mixture of mumbo-jumbo and strange potions. There is really no need for this attitude. The terms in use have developed for entirely valid reasons. They provide a degree of precision and a framework for diagnosis and decision-making. You should try to familiarize yourself with them and to apply them correctly. They will provide the building-blocks with which you will go on to make dermatological diagnoses. So, in the early days, describe everything you see in these terms as far as possible.

However, in most inflammatory dermatoses it is not always quite so simple because you have to decide *which lesion or lesions to select* for this descriptive process. Skin diseases are dynamic. In an eruption some lesions will be very early, some very late, and some at various intermediate evolutionary stages.

Try to examine as many patients as you can, because part of the value of frequent exposure to skin diseases is the development of an ability to recognize lesions which provide the most useful diagnostic information.

This diagnostic process will gradually become one which you perform increasingly easily and confidently as experience develops.

INVESTIGATION

Inevitably, history and examination alone will not always provide all the information required. There are some skin disorders in which further investigation is nearly always necessary: either to confirm a diagnosis with important prognostic or therapeutic implications (e.g. blistering disorders), or to seek an underlying, associated systemic disorder (e.g. in generalized pruritus). These situations are covered later in the appropriate chapters. Sometimes clinical findings alone will not produce a satisfactory working diagnosis, or further information is required in order to plan optimal management.

There are a number of important techniques which are available to provide further information. Some of these, such as appropriate blood tests and swabs for bacteriology and virology, should be familiar from other branches of medicine, and are fully covered in other introductory text-books. Others, however, are more specific to dermatological investigation. Common, useful investigations in skin diseases include the following:

INVESTIGATION TECHNIQUES

- Blood tests—for underlying systemic abnormalities
- Swabs—for infections
- Wood's light—some disorders/features are easier to see using this
- Skin scrapes or nail clips—microscopy and mycological culture
- Skin biopsy—histopathology; electron microscopy; immunopathology
- Patch tests—for evidence of contact allergy

Wood's light

This is a nickel oxide-filtered ultraviolet light. It is used to highlight three features of cutaneous disease:

I   certain organisms which cause scalp ringworm produce green fluorescence (useful in initial diagnosis and may be helpful in assessing the efficacy of therapy);

2 the organism responsible for erythrasma fluoresces coral-pink;

3 some pigmentary disorders are more clearly visible—particularly important are the pale patches seen in tuberous sclerosis, and café-au-lait marks in neurofibromatosis.

Wood's light can also be used to induce fluorescence in the urine in some of the porphyrias.

Scrapings/clippings

Material from the skin, hair or nails can be examined directly under the microscope and/or sent for culture. This is particularly useful in suspected fungal infection, molluscum contagiosum, or in a search for scabies mites (see Chapters 3–5). Scrapings are best taken with a 'banana' scalpel (which has a blunt, rather rounded blade). Scraping lightly will lift scales from the surface of the suspicious area.

The scales are placed on a microscope slide, covered with 10% potassium hydroxide (KOH) and a coverslip. After a few minutes to dissolve some of the epidermal cell membranes, they can be examined. It is helpful to add some ink if the organism being sought is *Pityrosporum* (the cause of pityriasis versicolor). Nail clippings can be treated in this manner, but need stronger solutions of KOH, or longer to dissolve, before examination.

Microscopy of hair may also provide information about fungal infections, may reveal structural hair shaft abnormalities in certain genetic disorders, and can be useful in distinguishing some causes of excessive hair loss (see Chapter 13).

Scrape/smear preparations are also used by some dermatologists for cytodiagnosis (Tzanck preparation) of suspected viral blisters and pemphigus. This technique enables material to be examined directly in the clinic, although very few dermatologists would rely on this alone.

Skin biopsy

Skin biopsy is a very important technique in the diagnosis of many skin disorders. In some, it is critical to have confirmation of a clinical diagnosis before embarking on treatment. Good examples of this are skin cancers, bullous disorders, and infections such as tuberculosis and leprosy. In others it is necessary to take a biopsy because clinical information alone has not provided all the answers.

There are two methods commonly used to obtain a skin sample for laboratory examination:

1 incisional/excisional biopsy;

2 punch biopsy.

INCISIONAL/EXCISIONAL BIOPSY

This provides good-sized samples (which can be divided for different purposes if required) and can be used to remove quite large lesions (see Figs 2.1 and 2.2)

1 Administer local anaesthetic
Usually 1–2% lignocaine; addition of 1 : 10 000 adrenaline helps reduce bleeding, but *never* use on extremities

2 For *incisional* (diagnostic) biopsy
Make two cuts forming an ellipse; ensure that the specimen is taken across the edge of the lesion, retaining a margin of normal perilesional skin (Fig. 2.1a)
For complete *excision*
Widen the ellipse around the whole lesion (Fig. 2.1b); ensure that the excision edge is cut vertically and does not slant in towards the tumour, as this can result in inadequate deeper excision (Fig. 2.3)

3 Repair the defect
Edges left by either incisional or excisional biopsy are brought neatly together with sutures; the choice of suture material is not critical, but for the best cosmetic result use the finest possible, preferably a synthetic monofilament suture (e.g. prolene)

Note: if there will be significant tension on the suture line, consider asking a trained plastic or dermatological surgeon for advice

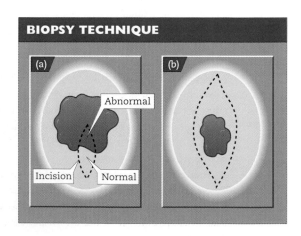

BIOPSY TECHNIQUE

Fig. 2.1 The technique for incisional/excisional biopsy.

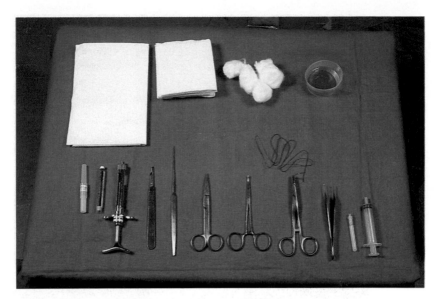

Fig. 2.2 Equipment needed for an incisional/excisional biopsy: sterile towel; gauze squares; cotton-wool balls; galley pot containing antiseptic; needle; cartridge of lignocaine and dental syringe; scalpel; skin hook; scissors; small artery forceps; needle holder and suture; fine, toothed forceps; needle and syringe (alternative to dental syringe).

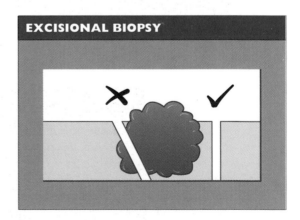

Fig. 2.3 Excisional biopsy: the correct (✓) and incorrect (×) excision edge.

Specimens obtained by either technique may be sent for conventional histopathology—normally fixed immediately in formal-saline—and/or other specialized examinations; for immunopathology the skin is usually snap frozen but for electron microscopy skin is best fixed in glutaraldehyde.

PUNCH BIOPSY

This is much quicker, but produces small samples and is only appropriate for diagnostic biopsies or removing tiny lesions (see Fig. 2.4a–c)

1 Administer local anaesthesia (see above)
2 Push the punch biopsy blade into the lesion using a circular motion
3 Lift out the small plug, and separate with scissors or a scalpel blade
4 Achieve haemostasis with silver nitrate or a small suture

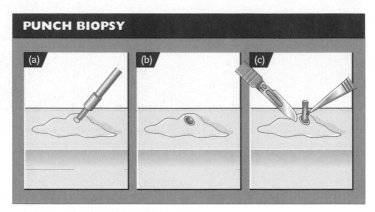

PUNCH BIOPSY

(a)   (b)   (c)

Fig. 2.4a–c The technique for a punch biopsy.

However, always check these details with the laboratory before you start.

Patch tests

If a contact allergic dermatitis is suspected, a patch test is performed. In this process possible allergens are usually diluted in suitable vehicles. The test materials are placed on inert tapes or in small discs (Fig. 2.5a,b), and then placed in contact with the skin (usually of the back) for 48 hours. A positive reaction (at 48 hours, or occasionally later) confirms a delayed hypersensitivity (Type IV) to the offending substance (Fig. 2.5c).

This technique can be extended to include testing for photoallergy.

CONCLUSION

You are now ready to start examining and talking to patients with skin disease. Attend some dermatology clinics and try to put these principles

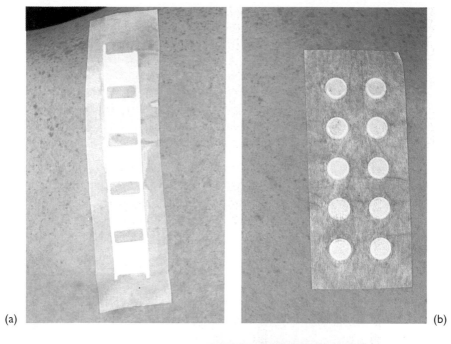

(a)

(b)

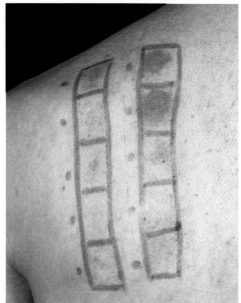

Fig. 2.5 Patch testing: (a) aluminium strip under tape; (b) metal cups under tape; (c) positive patch test reactions.

(c)

into practice. When seeing patients, try to retain a mental picture of their skin lesions. Ask the dermatologist in charge what the diagnosis is in each instance, and make sure that you read a little about each entity when the clinic is over.

The remaining chapters of this book are designed to help you to make specific diagnoses and to provide your patients with information about their problems, and to assist you in choosing appropriate treatment.

CHAPTER 3

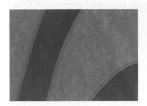

Bacterial and Viral Infections

A mighty creature is the germ,
Though smaller than the pachyderm.
His customary dwelling place
Is deep within the human race.
His childish pride he often pleases
By giving people strange diseases.
Do you, my poppet, feel infirm?
You probably contain a germ.
(Ogden Nash, *The Germ*)

BACTERIAL INFECTIONS

Streptococcal infection

CELLULITIS

Cellulitis is an infection of the skin and subcutaneous tissues by *Streptococcus pyogenes*. Superficial streptococcal infection of the skin is often called 'erysipelas', but a separate term seems unnecessary, as it is often impossible to judge the depth of tissue involved.

The legs are a common site for cellulitis, but other parts of the body, including the face, may be affected. The organisms probably gain entry into the skin via minor abrasions. A frequent predisposing factor is lower limb oedema, and cellulitis is a common condition in the elderly, who often

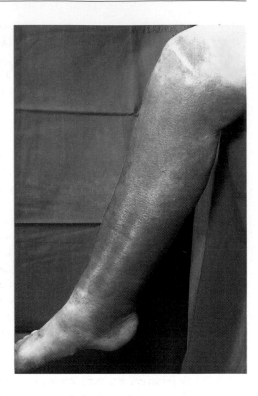

Fig. 3.1 Cellulitis.

suffer from leg oedema. Stasis ulcers provide a portal of entry for the organisms in some cases. The affected area becomes erythematous, hot, and swollen (Fig. 3.1), and occasionally blister formation and areas of skin necrosis occur. The patient is pyrexial and feels unwell. Rigors may occur, and, in the elderly, a toxic confusional state.

Strict bed rest is important in treatment. Cellulitis should be treated with parenteral penicillin. If extensive areas of tissue necrosis occur, surgical debridement may be necessary.

Some patients have recurrent episodes of cellulitis. Each episode damages lymphatics and leads to further oedema. These cases should be treated with prophylactic oral penicillin V or erythromycin, to prevent further cellulitic episodes.

Staphylococcal infection

FOLLICULITIS
Infection of the superficial part of a hair follicle with *Staphylococcus aureus*

produces a small pustule on an erythematous base, centred on the follicle. Folliculitis is a common problem in eczema patients treated with ointment-based topical steroid preparations.

Mild folliculitis can be treated with a topical antibacterial agent, but if extensive a systemic antibiotic may be required.

FURUNCULOSIS ('BOILS')

A boil is the result of deep infection of a hair follicle by *Staph. aureus*. A painful inflammatory nodule develops at the site of infection, and over a period of a few days becomes fluctuant and 'points' as a central pustule. Once the central necrotic core has been discharged, the lesion gradually resolves. In some patients boils are a recurrent problem, but this is rarely associated with a significant underlying disorder. Such individuals may be carriers of staphylococci in the nose, or on the perineum, and the organisms are transferred on the digits to various parts of the body.

Patients suffering from recurrent boils should have swabs taken from the nose for culture, and if found to be carrying staphylococci should be treated with a topical antibacterial such as mupirocin, applied to the nostrils. They may also be helped by an antibacterial bath additive, e.g. 2% triclosan, and a prolonged course of flucloxacillin.

CARBUNCLE

A carbuncle is a deep infection of a group of adjacent hair follicles with *Staph. aureus*. A frequent site for a carbuncle is the nape of the neck. Initially, the lesion is a dome-shaped area of tender erythema, but after a few days suppuration begins, and pus is discharged from multiple follicular orifices. Carbuncles are usually encountered in middle-aged and elderly men, and are frequently associated with diabetes or severe debility. Flucloxacillin should be given for treatment, and the abscesses drained.

IMPETIGO

This is a superficial infection caused by *Staph. aureus*, with or without haemolytic streptococci. Lesions may occur anywhere on the body. The initial lesion is a small pustule which rapidly increases in size, and ruptures to leave a raw, exuding surface. The exudate dries to form a golden-yellow crust, and the stratum corneum peels back at the margins of the affected area (Fig. 3.2). Impetigo may occur as a secondary phenomenon in atopic eczema, scabies and head louse infection.

Impetigo should generally be treated with a systemic antibiotic such as flucloxacillin or erythromycin. Useful topical antibacterial agents to use on localized cases, or as an adjunct to systemic therapy, are fusidic acid and mupirocin.

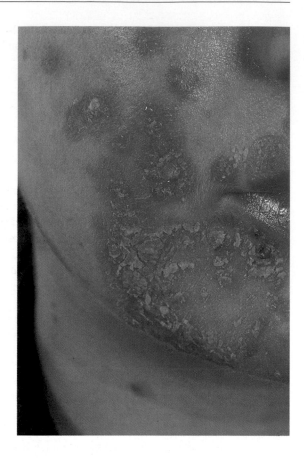

Fig. 3.2 Impetigo.

STAPHYLOCOCCAL SCALDED SKIN SYNDROME

This uncommon condition occurs as a result of infection with certain staphylococcal phage types which produce a toxin which splits the epidermis at the level of the granular layer. The superficial epidermis peels off in sheets, producing an appearance resembling scalded skin. Infants and young children are usually affected. It responds to treatment with flucloxacillin.

Erysipeloid

An infection with the organism *Erysipelothrix rhusiopathiae* may afflict those handling uncooked meat, poultry, fish and shellfish. It is therefore encountered in butchers, slaughterhouse workers, fishermen and fishmongers. The organism enters the skin via an abrasion, and produces a well-defined, purplish-red area which spreads gradually. There is no constitutional upset. It responds to treatment with penicillin.

Erythrasma

Caused by a Gram-positive bacillus, *Corynebacterium minutissimum*, erythrasma occurs in intertriginous areas—axillae, groins and sub-mammary regions. However, the commonest site colonized by this organism is the toe web-spaces, where it produces a macerated scaling appearance identical to that caused by fungal infection. In other sites it produces marginated brown areas with a fine, branny surface scale (Fig. 3.3). It is usually asymptomatic. *Corynebacterium minutissimum* produces a porphyrin which fluoresces a striking coral-pink under Wood's light.

Erythrasma may be treated with topical imidazoles (clotrimazole,

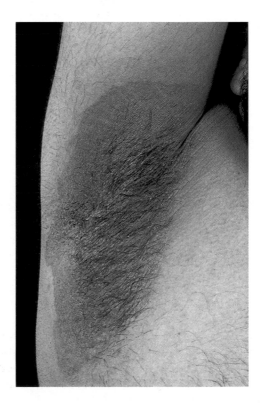

Fig. 3.3 Erythrasma in the axilla.

miconazole, econazole), topical fusidic acid, or a 2-week course of oral erythromycin.

Mycobacterial infection

CUTANEOUS TUBERCULOSIS

Cutaneous tuberculosis is now rare in the indigenous population of the UK, but is encountered in international residents, particularly those from the Indian subcontinent.

LUPUS VULGARIS

The lesions of lupus vulgaris are found on the head and neck in over 90% of cases. The typical appearance is of a reddish-brown, nodular plaque with a scaly surface (Fig. 3.4). When pressed with a glass slide (diascopy), the brown nodules are more easily seen, and are referred to as 'apple jelly nodules'. The natural course is gradual peripheral extension, and in many cases this is extremely slow. Active lupus vulgaris is a destructive process, and the cartilage of the nose and ears may be severely damaged.

Histology shows tubercles composed of epithelioid cells and Langhans' giant cells, usually without central caseation. Tubercle bacilli are present in very small numbers. The Mantoux test is strongly positive. The patient should be investigated for an underlying focus of tuberculosis in other organs, but this is only found in approximately 10% of cases.

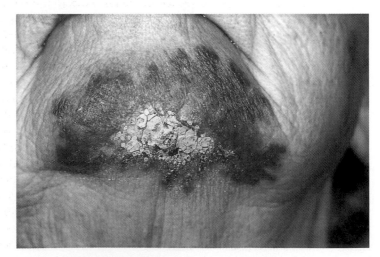

Fig. 3.4 Lupus vulgaris on the chin.

Treatment should be with standard anti-tuberculous chemotherapy. There is a risk of the development of squamous cell carcinoma in the scar tissue of long-standing lupus vulgaris.

WARTY TUBERCULOSIS

This is a chronic warty type of tuberculosis which occurs as a result of direct inoculation of tubercle bacilli into the skin of someone previously infected, who has a high degree of immunity. It may develop on the buttocks and thighs as a result of sitting on ground contaminated by infected sputum. It responds to standard anti-tuberculous chemotherapy.

TUBERCULIDES

This term is applied to a group of disorders which occur as an immunological response to tuberculosis elsewhere in the body. Included in this group are papulonecrotic tuberculide, lichen scrofulosorum and erythema induratum (Bazin's disease).

LEPROSY (HANSEN'S DISEASE)

The Norwegian Armauer Hansen discovered the leprosy bacillus, *Mycobacterium leprae*, in 1873. Leprosy has a wide distribution throughout the world, with the majority of cases occurring in the tropics and subtropics, but population movements mean that the disease may be encountered anywhere.

Leprosy is a disease of peripheral nerves, but it also affects the skin, and sometimes other tissues such as the eyes, the mucosa of the upper respiratory tract, the bones and the testes. Although it is infectious, the degree of infectivity is low. The incubation period is lengthy, probably several years, and it is likely that most patients acquire the infection in childhood. The disease is acquired as a result of close physical contact with an infected individual, the risk being much greater for contacts of lepromatous cases, but the portal of entry of the bacillus is unknown.

The clinical pattern of disease is determined by the host's cell-mediated immune response to the organism. When this is well developed tuberculoid leprosy occurs, in which skin and peripheral nerves are affected. Skin lesions are single, or few in number, and are well defined. They are macules or plaques which are hypopigmented in dark skin. The lesions are anaesthetic, sweating is absent, and hairs are reduced in number. Thickened branches of cutaneous sensory nerves may be palpable in the region of the lesions, and large peripheral nerves may also be palpable. The lepromin test is strongly positive. Histology shows well-defined tuberculoid granulomata, and bacilli are not seen on modified Ziehl–Nielsen staining.

When the cell-mediated immune response is poor, the bacilli multiply unchecked and the patient develops lepromatous leprosy. The bacilli spread to involve not only the skin, but also the mucosa of the respiratory tract, the eyes, testes and bones. Skin lesions are multiple and nodular. The lepromin test is negative. Histology shows a diffuse granuloma throughout the dermis, and bacilli are present in large numbers.

In between these two extreme, 'polar' forms of leprosy is a spectrum of disease referred to as borderline leprosy, the clinical and histological features of which reflect different degrees of cell-mediated response to the bacilli. There is no absolute diagnostic test for leprosy—the diagnosis is based on clinical and histological features.

Tuberculoid leprosy is usually treated with a combination of dapsone and rifampicin; lepromatous leprosy with dapsone, rifampicin and clofazimine. The treatment of leprosy may be complicated by immunologically mediated 'reactional states', and should be supervised by someone experienced in leprosy management.

THE LEPROSY SPECTRUM

Tuberculoid
- One or two skin lesions only
- Good cell-mediated immune response
- Positive lepromin test
- Few bacilli

Borderline
- Scattered skin lesions
- Intermediate cell-mediated immune response
- Some organisms

Lepromatous
- Extensive skin lesions and involvement of other organs
- Poor cell-mediated immune response
- Negative lepromin test
- Numerous organisms

ATYPICAL MYCOBACTERIA

The commonest of the skin lesions produced by atypical mycobacteria is 'swimming pool' or 'fish tank' granuloma. This is usually a solitary granulomatous nodule, caused by inoculation of *Mycobacterium marinum* into the skin via an abrasion sustained whilst swimming, or in tropical fish fanciers whilst cleaning out the aquarium. Occasionally, in addition to the initial lesion, there are multiple secondary lesions in a linear distribution along the lines of lymphatics (sporotrichoid spread). Conventional anti-tuberculous chemotherapy is often not very effective, but minocycline or co-trimoxazole are usually curative.

VIRAL INFECTIONS

Warts

Fasting spittle is good for warts. (Traditional English)

Warts are benign epidermal neoplasms caused by viruses of the human papillomavirus (HPV) group. There are a number of different strains of HPV which produce different clinical types of warts. Warts are also known as 'verrucae', although the term verruca in popular usage is usually reserved for the plantar wart.

COMMON WARTS

These are raised, cauliflower-like lesions which occur most frequently on the hands. They are extremely common in childhood and early adult life. They may be scattered, grouped or periungual in distribution. Common warts in children usually resolve spontaneously.

Common warts are usually treated with wart paints or cryotherapy. Preparations containing salicylic acid, glutaraldehyde, or formaldehyde are often quite effective, and a wart paint should certainly be used for at least 3 months before considering alternative treatment.

Cryotherapy with liquid nitrogen can be used on resistant warts. A simple applicator of cotton wool on the end of an orange stick is dipped in the nitrogen and applied to the wart until it and a narrow rim of surrounding skin are frozen. It is a painful procedure, and should not be inflicted on small children. Multiple warts usually require more than one application, and the optimum interval between treatments is 2–3 weeks.

PLANTAR WARTS

Plantar warts may be solitary, scattered over the sole of the foot, or grouped together producing so-called mosaic warts (Fig. 3.5). The typical appearance is of a small area of thickened skin which, when pared away, reveals several black dots produced by thrombosed capillaries. Plantar warts are frequently painful. They must be distinguished from calluses and corns, which develop in areas of friction over bony prominences. Calluses are patches of uniformly thickened skin, and corns have a painful central plug of keratin which does not contain capillaries.

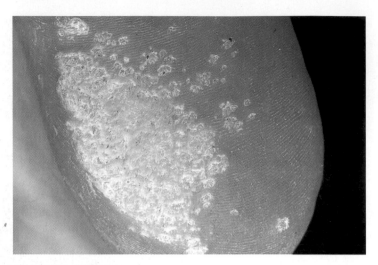

Fig. 3.5 Mosaic plantar warts.

Wart paints are the mainstay of treatment for plantar warts— cryotherapy is not as effective as it is on hand warts.

PLANE WARTS

These are tiny, flat-topped, flesh-coloured warts which usually occur on the dorsa of the hands and the face (Fig. 3.6). They often occur in lines due to inoculation of the virus into scratches and abrasions. Plane warts are extremely difficult to treat effectively, and attempts at treatment may do more harm than good. They will resolve spontaneously eventually, and are best left alone.

GENITAL WARTS (CONDYLOMATA ACUMINATA)

In recent years the importance of certain types of genital wart viruses in the aetiology of penile and cervical cancer has been recognized, and this has modified attitudes to what was previously considered a minor sexually transmitted inconvenience. It is now more appropriate that patients suffering from genital warts are seen and treated in a department of genitourinary medicine, so that coexisting sexually transmitted disease may be detected, and sexual contacts traced and examined.

MOLLUSCUM CONTAGIOSUM

The lesions of molluscum contagiosum are caused by a pox virus. They are typically pearly, pink papules with a central umbilication filled with a horny

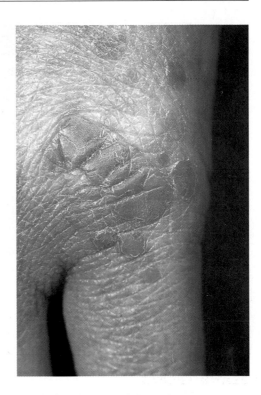

Fig. 3.6 Plane warts.

plug (Fig. 3.7). The lesions may occur anywhere on the body, but are most common on the head and neck area and the trunk. They are frequently grouped, and may be surrounded by a mild eczematous reaction. They may be very extensive in children with atopic eczema.

No antiviral agent has any effect on the virus causing these lesions, but their natural history is of spontaneous resolution. In infants and young children they are best left to resolve spontaneously, but if parents are anxious they can be advised to squeeze each lesion between the thumbnails to express the central plug—this will often speed their resolution. In older children and adults molluscum contagiosum can be treated by cryotherapy.

ORF

Orf is a viral disease of sheep which can be transmitted to humans. Those usually affected are women who bottle-feed lambs, and butchers and slaughterhouse workers who handle the carcasses of sheep. The typical clinical picture is of a solitary, inflammatory papule which rapidly develops into a domed nodule of granulation tissue—usually on a finger (Fig. 3.8)—

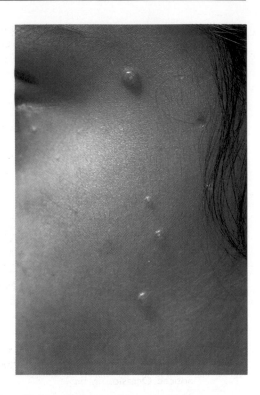

Fig. 3.7 Molluscum
contagiosum.

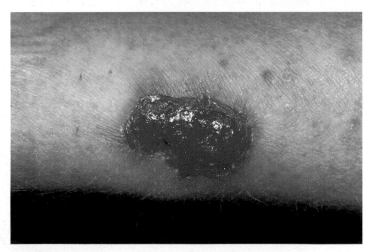

Fig. 3.8 Orf.

but occasionally on the face. Rarely there are multiple lesions. The diagnosis can be confirmed by electron microscopy of smears from the granulation tissue. Orf lesions resolve spontaneously in 6–8 weeks. Orf may act as a trigger for erythema multiforme.

HAND, FOOT AND MOUTH DISEASE

This disease is produced by Coxsackie virus infection, usually type A16. Small greyish vesicles with a halo of erythema occur on the hands and feet (Fig. 3.9), and the buccal mucosa is studded with erosions resembling aphthous ulcers. The condition resolves within 2 weeks and no treatment is required.

Herpes simplex

There are two antigenic types of the herpes simplex virus. Type 1 is responsible for the common 'cold sore' on the lips and face, and Type 2 is associated with genital herpes. Neither has rigid territorial demarcation, however, and lesions anywhere may be caused by either antigenic type.

PRIMARY HERPES SIMPLEX

Initial contact with the herpes simplex virus usually occurs in early childhood, and any lesions which develop are often so mild that they are not noticed. Occasionally, however, a severe primary herpetic gingivostomatitis occurs, with painful erosions on the buccal mucosa and lips. Primary

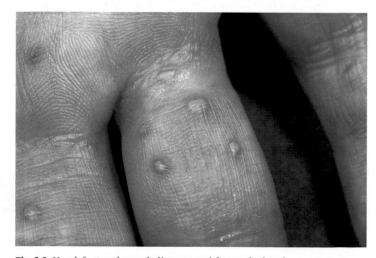

Fig. 3.9 Hand, foot and mouth disease: vesicles on the hand.

cutaneous herpes simplex may also occur, and in atopic eczema this can be very extensive and may be life-threatening (see below).

Following a primary infection the virus settles in sensory ganglia, and may be triggered to produce recurrent lesions by a variety of stimuli.

RECURRENT HERPES SIMPLEX

Recurrent cold sores on the lips (herpes labialis) are common. A group of small vesicles is preceded by itching and discomfort in the affected area. The vesicles subsequently burst, the lesion crusts over, and usually resolves in 10–14 days. The trigger for these episodes is often fever, but exposure to strong sunlight, and menses, are also recognized precipitants. Occasionally, as a result of inoculation of the virus into a finger, painful episodes of 'herpetic whitlow' occur. The frequency of episodes of herpes simplex usually gradually declines with advancing age.

Labial herpes simplex is usually a minor cosmetic inconvenience, and does not require treatment. However, if episodes are frequent and troublesome, topical aciclovir may be of benefit. This blocks viral replication—it is not viricidal, and is not curative.

HERPES SIMPLEX AND ERYTHEMA MULTIFORME

Recurrent herpes simplex can trigger episodes of erythema multiforme. Prophylactic oral aciclovir may be of considerable benefit in the management of severe cases.

ECZEMA HERPETICUM (KAPOSI'S VARICELLIFORM ERUPTION)

This is a widespread herpes simplex infection which occurs in atopic eczema. The head and neck are frequently affected, but lesions may spread rapidly to involve extensive areas of skin (Fig. 3.10). Lymphadenopathy and constitutional upset may occur. If the disease is limited in distribution and the patient is seen early in its course, oral aciclovir therapy is appropriate. However, if the lesions are extensive, and the patient is unwell, they should be admitted to hospital and treated with intravenous aciclovir. Topical steroid therapy should be stopped until the herpes has resolved. Secondary bacterial infection is common, and a systemic antibiotic should be given. Eczema herpeticum may recur, but subsequent episodes tend to be less severe.

Herpes zoster (shingles)

Chicken-pox and herpes zoster are both caused by the varicella zoster virus, which is similar in size and structure to the herpes simplex virus. *Shingles* is a distortion of the Latin *cingulum*, meaning a girdle.

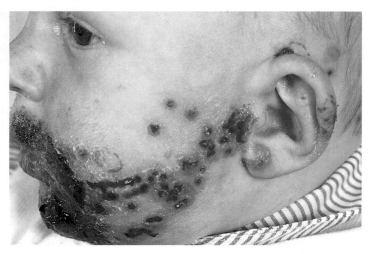

Fig. 3.10 Eczema herpeticum.

Following an attack of chicken-pox the virus remains dormant in dorsal root ganglia until some stimulus reactivates it and causes an attack of shingles. The middle-aged and elderly are most often affected, but it occasionally occurs in childhood. It is also more frequent in immunosuppressed individuals.

Shingles usually affects a single dermatome, most commonly on the thorax or abdomen. The eruption may be preceded by pain in the region of the dermatome, and this occasionally leads to an incorrect diagnosis of internal pathology. The lesions consist of a unilateral band of grouped vesicles on an erythematous base (Fig. 3.11). The contents of the vesicles are initially clear, but subsequently become cloudy. There may be scattered outlying vesicles on the rest of the body, and these tend to be more numerous in the elderly. Numerous outlying vesicles (disseminated zoster) are also seen in immunosuppressed individuals. After a few days the vesicles dry up and form crusts, and in most cases the eruption resolves within 2 weeks.

However, in the elderly, shingles may produce erosive changes which take considerably longer to heal. There is usually some residual scarring. The most troublesome aspect of shingles is the persistence of pain after the lesions have resolved (postherpetic neuralgia). This may be very severe, and is particularly distressing for the elderly.

Sacral zoster

Sacral zoster may cause acute retention of urine.

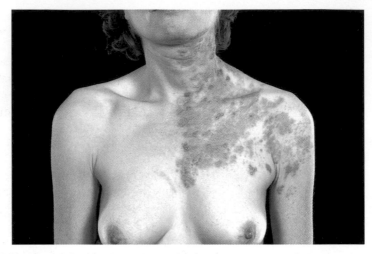

Fig. 3.11 Herpes zoster.

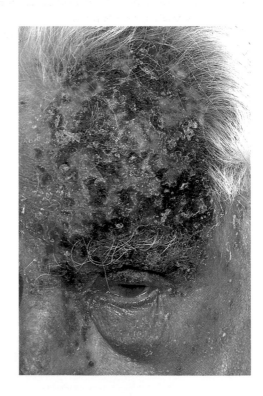

Fig. 3.12 Ophthalmic zoster.

Trigeminal zoster

Herpes zoster may affect any of the divisions of the trigeminal nerve, but the ophthalmic division is most frequently involved (Fig. 3.12). Ocular problems such as conjunctivitis, keratitis and/or iridocyclitis may occur if the nasociliary branch of the ophthalmic division is affected, and patients with ophthalmic zoster should be examined by an ophthalmologist.

Involvement of the maxillary division of the trigeminal nerve produces vesicles on the cheek, and unilateral vesicles on the palate.

Motor zoster

Occasionally, in addition to skin lesions in a sensory dermatome, motor fibres are affected, leading to muscle paralysis and subsequent atrophy.

TREATMENT OF HERPES ZOSTER

Most cases do not require any treatment. However, in severe cases, oral aciclovir may be of benefit. In disseminated zoster in the immunosuppressed, intravenous aciclovir can be life-saving, and it may also be useful in cases of ophthalmic zoster.

Pain relief is often difficult to achieve in postherpetic neuralgia, and patients with severe discomfort should be referred to a pain relief specialist.

CHAPTER 4

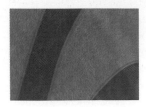

Fungal Infections

The fungi which may cause human disease include the *dermatophytes* (Greek, meaning 'skin plants') and the yeast-like fungus *Candida albicans*, which are responsible for superficial fungal infections confined to the skin and mucous membranes. Other fungi can invade living tissue to cause deep infections, which may remain localized (mycetoma) or cause systemic disease (e.g. histoplasmosis).

The dermatophytes are a group of fungi responsible for so-called 'ringworm' infections. The vegetative phase of dermatophyte fungi consists of septate hyphae which form a branching network (mycelium). *Candida albicans* is an organism composed of round or oval cells which divide by budding. Apart from its yeast form it may produce pseudohyphae consisting of numerous cells in a linear arrangement or, in certain circumstances, true septate hyphae.

DERMATOPHYTE INFECTIONS

It is easy to become totally confused by the terminology used in relation to fungal infection. Hence, it is advisable for the novice not to attempt to learn the names of fungi. The term 'ringworm', followed by 'of the feet, of the groin, of the scalp' etc., is a simple way of indicating the location of the infection. If you feel in more classical mood you may use 'tinea' (Latin meaning 'a gnawing worm') followed by 'pedis, cruris, capitis' etc. The fungi are named according to their genus (*Microsporum, Trichophyton* and *Epidermophyton*) and species (e.g. *Microsporum canis, Trichophyton rubrum*), and they can be distinguished from one another in culture. An experienced dermatologist may be able to suggest that a certain fungus is responsible for a particular case of ringworm, but the only way to establish its identity precisely is by culture.

Some fungi are confined to humans (anthropophilic), others principally affect animals (zoophilic) but occasionally infect humans. When animal fungi cause human skin lesions their presence usually provokes a severe inflammatory reaction. Dermatophytes grow only in keratin—the stratum corneum of the skin, hair, and nails. Infection is usually acquired by contact with keratin debris carrying fungal hyphae.

TINEA PEDIS (ATHLETE'S FOOT)

This is the commonest of the dermatophyte infections, and usually presents as scaling, itchy areas in the toe webs, particularly between the fourth and fifth toes (Fig. 4.1). It is usually acquired from contact with infected keratin debris on the floors of swimming-pools and showers. The condition may spread onto the soles or the dorsa of the feet as areas of scaling erythema. Occasionally, athlete's foot follows a pattern of episodic vesicular lesions on the soles of the feet, occurring particularly during

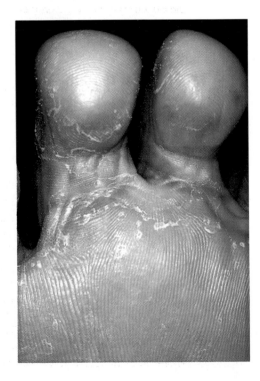

Fig. 4.1 Athlete's foot.

warm weather. The feet are frequently asymmetrically involved in fungal infection, in contrast with eczema, in which the involvement is usually symmetrical.

TINEA CRURIS

This is common in men and rare in women. The clinical picture is characteristic, and should be easy to distinguish from intertrigo, flexural psoriasis or flexural seborrhoeic dermatitis. A scaly, erythematous margin gradually spreads down the medial aspects of the thighs (Fig. 4.2), and may extend to involve the perineum and buttocks. The source of the infection is almost always the patient's feet, so they should be examined for evidence of athlete's foot or fungal nail dystrophy. The fungus is transferred to the groins on the fingers or on towels.

TINEA CORPORIS

The lesions are typically annular, with a scaly inflammatory edge and central clearing (Fig. 4.3). In children the organism is usually of animal

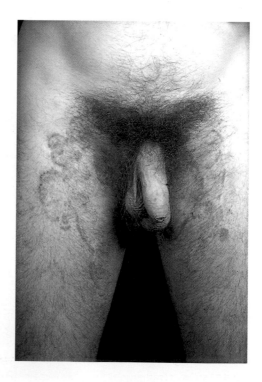

Fig. 4.2 Tinea cruris.

origin—most frequently a kitten. In adults the fungus is spread from the feet or groins.

TINEA MANUUM

Ringworm on the hand is usually unilateral. On the palm of the hand the appearance is of mild scaling erythema, whereas on the dorsum there is more obvious inflammatory change, with a well-defined edge (Fig. 4.4).

TINEA UNGUIUM

Toenail fungal dystrophy is very common in adults, and is invariably associated with athlete's foot. The involvement usually starts distally as yellowish streaks in the nail plate (Fig. 4.5), but gradually the whole nail becomes thickened, discoloured and friable. The great toenails are often the first to be involved, and pressure from footwear on the thickened nails may produce considerable discomfort.

Fingernails are less commonly affected. The changes in the nail plate are similar to those seen in toenails (Fig. 4.6).

TINEA CAPITIS

Tinea capitis is principally a disease of childhood, and is rare in adults. This is thought to be related to a change in the fatty acid constituents of sebum

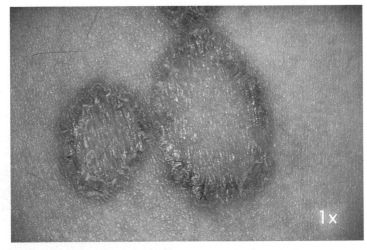

Fig. 4.3 Tinea corporis in a child (*Microsporum canis*—from a cat).

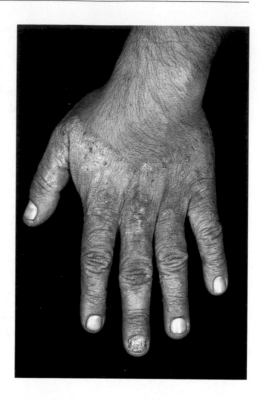

Fig. 4.4 Tinea on the dorsum of the hand.

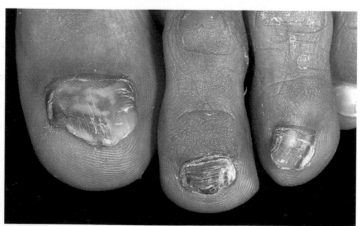

Fig. 4.5 Tinea of the toenails.

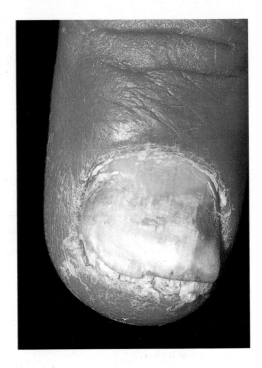

Fig. 4.6 Tinea of a fingernail.

around the time of puberty. Post-pubertal sebum contains fungistatic fatty acids. The principal fungi responsible for scalp ringworm vary in different parts of the world. In the UK, most cases of scalp ringworm in the indigenous population are the result of *M. canis* infection, usually acquired from cats, and in the USA the usual causative organism is *Trichophyton tonsurans*. In the Indian subcontinent the commonest cause is a fungus called *Trichophyton violaceum*.

One or more patches of partial hair loss develop on an otherwise normal scalp (Fig. 4.7), but occasionally the involvement is more extensive, producing an appearance suggestive of seborrhoeic dermatitis. The affected scalp is scaly, and the hair is usually broken off just above the surface, producing an irregular stubble. Some fungi, for example *M. canis*, fluoresce yellow–green under long wavelength ultraviolet (UV) light (Wood's light)—see Chapter 2.

KERION

Kerion (Greek meaning 'honeycomb') is a term applied to severe inflammatory scalp ringworm, usually provoked by the fungus of cattle ringworm,

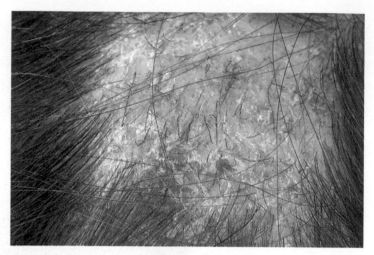

Fig. 4.7 Scalp ringworm.

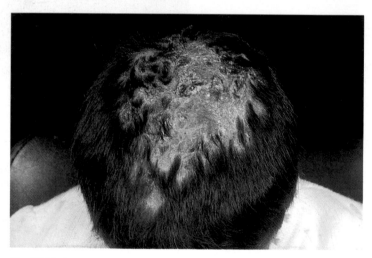

Fig. 4.8 Kerion.

but occasionally by other fungi. It resembles a bacterial infection, with pustules and abscesses (Fig. 4.8), but bacterial culture is negative. There may be areas of permanent hair loss.

CATTLE RINGWORM

In rural areas, young farm workers often suffer from cattle ringworm—older farmers have usually had the disease—and develop immunity against

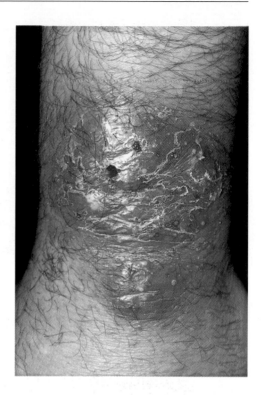

Fig. 4.9 Cattle ringworm on the forearm of a farmer.

re-infection. Children who visit farms may pick up the fungus from gates and fences where cattle have left keratin debris containing the organism. In adults, the face and forearms are the areas most frequently affected (Fig. 4.9). In children the scalp is the usual site of infection, and the fungus provokes a kerion.

TINEA INCOGNITO

This term is applied to a fungal infection whose appearance has been altered by inappropriate treatment with topical steroid preparations. Topical steroids suppress the inflammatory response to the fungus, and the typical scaly erythematous margin may disappear, leaving an ill-defined area studded with pustules.

'Ide' reactions

Patients suffering from the florid vesicular type of athlete's foot may develop an acute vesiculo-bullous eruption on the hands, known as an 'ide'

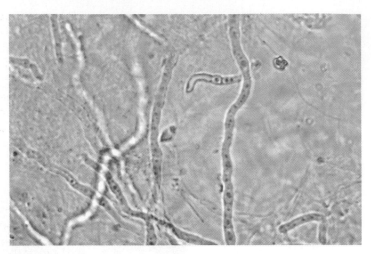

Fig. 4.10 Fungal mycelium.

reaction. The lesions on the hands do not contain fungus. The reaction appears to have an immunological basis, but the exact pathomechanism is unknown. Occasionally, a more generalized maculopapular ide reaction accompanies a fungal infection.

Diagnosis

Skin scrapings, nail clippings and plucked hair can be examined as described in Chapter 2. A little experience is necessary to distinguish fungal mycelium (Fig. 4.10) from cell walls and intercellular lipid, or filamentous debris. Fungal mycelium has the appearance of long rows of railway wagons which branch periodically. Material should also be sent to the mycology laboratory for culture.

Treatment

There are a number of broad-spectrum topical antifungal agents available for the treatment of dermatophyte infections, including miconazole, clotrimazole, econazole, sulconazole and terbinafine. These can be used when small areas of skin are affected, but if a fungal infection is extensive it is preferable to employ an oral agent such as griseofulvin, itraconazole or terbinafine. Topical agents are not effective in scalp ringworm, and this should be treated with griseofulvin. For skin and hair infections griseofulvin should be given for a period of 4–6 weeks. In children the dosage is calculated according to the child's weight; in adults the usual daily dose is

500 mg. Skin infections may also be treated with itraconazole 100 mg daily for 15–30 days, or terbinafine 250 mg daily for 4 weeks.

For many years griseofulvin was used to treat dermatophyte infection of the nails, but the duration of treatment is lengthy—6 months for fingernails and 18 months for toenails. It is quite effective in fingernail infections, but the cure rate for toenails is much lower. Terbinafine is now the treatment of choice for nail dermatophyte infections. The recommended regimen for fingernails is 250 mg daily for 6 weeks, and for toenails treatment should be continued for 3 months. Cure rates are significantly higher than those obtained with griseofulvin.

Mycetoma (Madura foot)

In certain parts of the world, for example the Indian subcontinent, trauma to the feet may result in the inoculation of certain soil fungi, which produce a chronic infection with abscesses and draining sinuses.

CANDIDA INFECTION

Candidiasis (moniliasis; 'thrush') is a term applied to infections of the skin and mucous membranes by yeast-like fungi of the genus *Candida*. The commonest, *Candida albicans*, is a normal commensal of the human digestive tract, where it exists in balance with the bacterial flora. In its commensal role, *Candida* is present as budding yeasts. In a pathogenic role, budding and mycelial forms are usually present. It only becomes pathogenic when situations favourable to its multiplication arise. These include topical and systemic steroid therapy, immune suppression of any aetiology, broad-spectrum antibiotics, diabetes mellitus, and the apposition of areas of skin to produce a warm, moist environment.

The diagnosis of candidiasis can be confirmed by culture of swabs taken from the affected areas.

BUCCAL MUCOSAL CANDIDIASIS

White, curd-like plaques adhere to the buccal mucosa. If these are scraped off, the underlying epithelium is inflamed and friable. It may be treated with nystatin oral suspension, amphotericin lozenges, or miconazole gel.

ANGULAR CHEILITIS (PERLÈCHE)

As we age, the vertical dimensions of the face gradually diminish. This may produce deep grooves at the angles of the mouth. Saliva is drawn into these grooves by capillary action, and enzymes macerate the skin, producing sore, moist areas (Fig. 4.11). *Candida* from the mouth multiplies in these conditions, and exacerbates the problem. Most patients with this problem

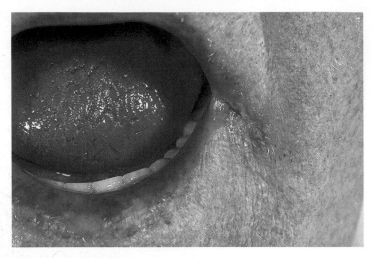

Fig. 4.11 Angular cheilitis.

are denture wearers, and modification of the dentures may help. The topical application of nystatin or an imidazole antifungal (clotrimazole, miconazole, econazole) will also help. Occasionally, angular cheilitis is a feature of iron or vitamin B_{12} deficiency, and it is advisable to perform a full blood count.

CHRONIC PARONYCHIA

This is a chronic inflammatory process affecting the proximal nail fold and nail matrix. *Candida albicans* plays a pathogenic role, but bacteria may also be involved. The condition is quite distinct from acute staphylococcal paronychia, in which there is a short history, severe discomfort, and ample production of green pus. The appearance in chronic paronychia is of thickening and erythema of the proximal nail fold ('bolstering'), and loss of the cuticle (Fig. 4.12). There is often an associated nail dystrophy. Chronic paronychia occurs predominantly in those whose hands are repeatedly immersed in water—housewives, barstaff, florists, fishmongers.

Treatment consists of advice to keep the hands as dry as possible by wearing cotton-lined rubber or PVC gloves when working, and topical anti-*Candida* therapy.

BALANITIS/VULVOVAGINITIS

Small white patches or eroded areas are present on the foreskin and glans of the uncircumcised. Predisposing factors are poor penile hygiene, and diabetes mellitus. *Candida* balanitis may be a recurrent problem if a sexual

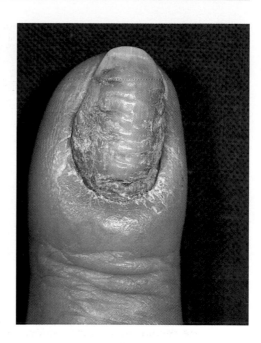

Fig. 4.12 Chronic paronychia.

partner has *Candida* vaginitis.

Candida vulvovaginitis presents with a creamy vaginal discharge and itchy erythema of the vulva. Pregnancy, oral contraceptives and diabetes mellitus are predisposing factors.

Balanitis and vulvitis should be treated with a topical anti-*Candida* preparation, and there are several products available to treat vaginal candidiasis.

Don't forget to test the urine for sugar in anyone with *Candida* balanitis or vulvovaginitis.

INTERTRIGO

'Intertrigo' is a term applied to maceration which occurs where two skin surfaces are in apposition—groins, axillae, sub-mammary regions—beneath an abdominal fat apron. Obesity and poor hygiene are contributory factors. *Candida* superinfection is often present, and is suggested clinically by the presence of creamy 'satellite' pustules at the margins of the affected areas. The pustules are easily ruptured, leaving a collarette of scale. This gives a characteristic scalloped edge to the area of intertrigo.

Therapy with a combination of an anti-*Candida* agent and hydrocortisone is usually beneficial, but attention to hygiene is also important.

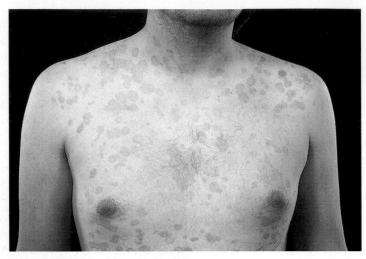

Fig. 4.13 Pityriasis versicolor.

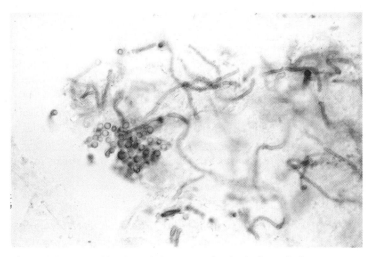

Fig. 4.14 Spores and hyphae of *Pityrosporum* in pityriasis versicolor.

PITYRIASIS (TINEA) VERSICOLOR

This is a common condition in young adults, and is caused by yeast-like organisms (*Pityrosporum* species), which are normal skin commensals present in pilosebaceous follicles. An alteration in the microenvironment encourages them to multiply and extend on to the surface of the skin.

On a non-pigmented skin, the lesions are light-brown macules with a fine surface scale, and they occur predominantly on the trunk and upper arms (Fig. 4.13). They are usually asymptomatic. On a pigmented skin, the typical appearance is of patchy hypopigmentation.

The diagnosis can be confirmed by microscopic examination of skin scrapings in a mixture of 10% potassium hydroxide and Parker Quink ink (Fig. 4.14), when characteristic clumps of round spores and short, stubby hyphae can be seen ('spaghetti and meat balls').

A simple treatment is selenium sulphide, in the form of a shampoo, left on the skin for a few minutes during bathing. This will usually clear the organism in 2–3 weeks. Broad-spectrum topical antifungal agents, or a 7-day course of oral itraconazole, are also effective against this organism. Griseofulvin is not. Tinea versicolor tends to recur, and treatment may have to be repeated. Hypopigmented areas may take a considerable time to re-pigment, and their persistence should not be taken as evidence of treatment failure.

CHAPTER 5

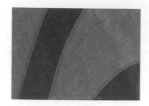

Ectoparasite Infections

SCABIES

There's a squeak of pure delight from a matey little mite,
As it tortuously tunnels in the skin,
Singing furrow, folly furrow, come and join me in my burrow,
And we'll view the epidermis from within.
                   (Guy's *Acarus*)

AETIOLOGY

Scabies (Latin *scabere*—to scratch) is caused by the mite *Sarcoptes scabiei*, and is acquired by close physical contact with someone suffering from the disease—sexual contact is often implicated but prolonged hand holding is probably a frequent means of spread. Any age group may be affected, but it is commoner in children and young adults. Transient contact is not sufficient for spread, and doctors and nurses who encounter ordinary cases of scabies should not be afraid of acquiring the disease.

    The female scabies mite burrows in the epidermis, and lays eggs in the burrow behind her. Initially, the host is unaware of the mining activity in the epidermis, but after a period of 4–6 weeks hypersensitivity to mite faeces develops, and itching begins. Thereafter, burrows will be excoriated and mites and eggs destroyed. In this way the host keeps the mite population in check, and in most individuals suffering from scabies the average number of adult female mites on the skin is no more than a dozen.

CLINICAL FEATURES

The patient complains of itching, which is characteristically worse at night. Scabies should be considered in anyone presenting with this history.

There are two principal types of skin lesion in scabies—burrows and the scabies 'rash'. Burrows are found principally on the hands and feet—the sides of the fingers and toes, the web-spaces, the wrists, and the insteps. In infants, burrows are often present on the palms of the hands and soles of the feet, and may also be present on the trunk. Burrows on the trunk are also a common finding in the elderly. Each burrow is several millimetres long, usually tortuous, light-brown in colour, and often surrounded by mild erythema (Fig. 5.1). Burrows also occur on the male genitalia, usually surmounting an inflammatory papule, and these lesions are pathognomonic of scabies. If scabies is suspected in a male, the genitalia should always be examined.

The 'rash' of scabies is an eruption of tiny inflammatory papules grouped on the axillary folds, around the umbilicus, and on the thighs (Fig. 5.2). The aetiology of these papules is not known with certainty, but they are thought to occur as a reaction to burrowing immature mites.

In addition to these primary skin lesions, there may be secondary changes such as excoriations, eczematization and secondary bacterial infection. In some tropical countries, secondary bacterial infection is extremely common.

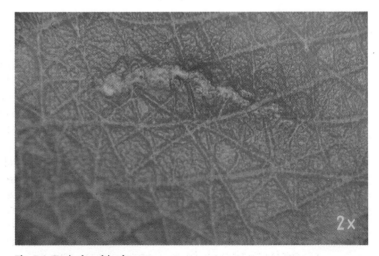

Fig. 5.1 Typical scabies burrow.

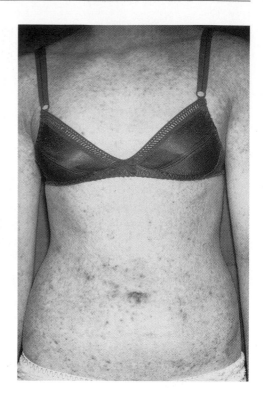

Fig. 5.2 The scabies 'rash'.

DIAGNOSIS

Absolute confirmation of the diagnosis can only be made by demonstrating the mites or eggs microscopically. In order to do this, burrows must be found, and this usually requires some expertise. Look carefully, in good light, at the hands and feet. A magnifying glass may be of some help, but myopia is a distinct advantage. Once a burrow, or suspected burrow, has been identified, it should be gently scraped off the skin with the edge of a blunt scalpel—dermatologists often use a 'banana' scalpel for this task (see Chapter 2). The burrow and its contents should be placed on a microscope slide with a few drops of 10% potassium hydroxide, covered with a coverslip, and examined under the microscope. The presence of mites, eggs, or even egg-shells confirms the diagnosis (Fig. 5.3).

Do not attempt to scrape lesions on the penis—the proximity of a banana scalpel to the nether regions leads to understandable

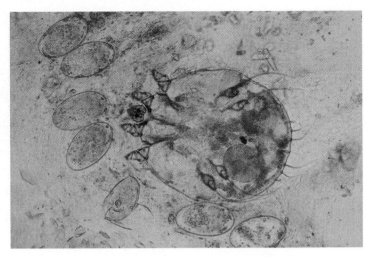

Fig. 5.3 Scabies mite and eggs in potassium hydroxide preparation.

apprehension, and is in any case rarely rewarded by the demonstration of mites.

TREATMENT

Scabies is treated by eating young alligators and washing the skin with urine. (Mexican Folk Medicine)

It is important to explain to patients precisely how to use their treatment, and written explanatory treatment sheets are useful. All family members, and close physical contacts of an affected individual, should be treated simultaneously. Liquid preparations should be applied from the neck to the toes, using a 2-inch paint brush. Itching does not resolve immediately following treatment, but will improve gradually over 2–3 weeks as the superficial epidermis, containing the allergenic mite faeces, is shed. A topical antipruritic such as Eurax-Hydrocortisone cream (crotamiton 10% and hydrocortisone 0.25%) can be used on residual itchy areas. It is not necessary to 'disinfest' clothing and soft furnishings—laundering of underwear and nightclothes is all that is required.

Available treatments

These are as follows:

> ### TREATMENTS
>
> **Benzyl benzoate emulsion**
> Three applications in a 24-hour period are usually sufficient. On the evening of day 1 apply the emulsion from the neck to the toes. Allow to dry, then apply a second coat. The following morning apply a third coat, and then wash off the benzyl benzoate on the evening of day 2. Treatment is then complete, and this should be stressed to the patient, because benzyl benzoate is an irritant, and repeated use will produce an irritant dermatitis
>
> **Lindane lotion**
> Leave on the skin for 12–24 hours, and then wash off. Repeat if necessary after 7 days
>
> **Monosulfiram solution**
> Dilute with two to three parts of water before application. Wash off after 24 hours
>
> **Aqueous malathion**
> Wash off after 24 hours. A second application may be necessary after 5–7 days
>
> **5% permethrin cream**
> Wash off after 8–24 hours

Scabies mites rarely burrow on the head and neck, except in infants, and it is not necessary to treat these areas.

Treatment of infants and young children

Benzyl benzoate is an irritant, and should be diluted to half-strength if used to treat infants. Any of the other agents listed can be used in the treatment of young children, although there is some debate about lindane, as there have been reports of transient neurological problems following its use on infants. The experience of most dermatologists is that it is safe if used correctly.

If burrows are present on the head and neck area in babies, these can be treated with topical Eurax (crotamiton 10%) cream.

NORWEGIAN (CRUSTED) SCABIES

This is a rare type of scabies in which enormous numbers of mites are present in crusted lesions on the skin. It is called Norwegian scabies because it was originally described in Norwegian lepers—the mite is exactly the same as that causing ordinary scabies. Mites are present in such huge numbers because of an altered host response to their presence. Norwegian scabies may develop when itching is not perceived because of mental abnormality, sensory loss from neurological disorders, or when the hypersensitivity response to the parasites is reduced by immunosuppressive therapy. Patients who are physically incapacitated may also develop crusted scabies because they are unable to scratch, and the mite population therefore multiplies unchecked.

The hyperkeratotic skin lesions in Norwegian scabies contain thousands of mites and eggs, and these are shed into the environment on flakes of keratin. Anyone coming into contact with a patient suffering from crusted scabies is at risk of acquiring ordinary scabies, and undiagnosed cases may be responsible for outbreaks of scabies in hospitals and residential homes.

CLINICAL FEATURES

The hands and feet are usually encased in a thick, fissured crust, and areas of crusting may be present on other parts of the body. The changes may resemble psoriatic scaling or a hyperkeratotic eczema, and this is why the diagnosis may be missed. Burrows are usually impossible to identify in the crusted areas, but may be found on less severely affected parts of the body. Microscopy of scales reveals numerous mites and eggs.

TREATMENT

The patient should be isolated, and nurses responsible for their care should wear gowns and gloves. All nursing and medical staff who have been in contact with the patient, and all other individuals who share the same accommodation, should be treated with a topical scabicide.

Crusted scabies usually requires several applications of a scabicide to eradicate the problem.

PEDICULOSIS

Head lice (*Pediculus humanus capitis*)

Her ladyship said when I went to her house,
That she did not esteem me three skips of a louse;
I freely forgave what the dear creature said,
For ladies will talk of what runs in their head.
            (Theodore Hook)

Head lice are wingless insects which live on the scalp, and feed on blood. Adult head lice are approximately 2–3 mm in length. They are acquired by head-to-head contact with another infected individual. It is unlikely that fomites, such as caps, brushes and combs, are responsible for transmission of the head louse. In the past, head louse infection was principally a problem of the lower classes in large industrial conurbations, but in recent years the head louse has climbed the social ladder and is now a common problem in all social classes.

The adult female louse lays eggs which she cements to hair shafts (Fig. 5.4). The eggs are flesh-coloured and are difficult to see, but once the louse nymph has emerged the empty egg-case (nit) is more readily visible.

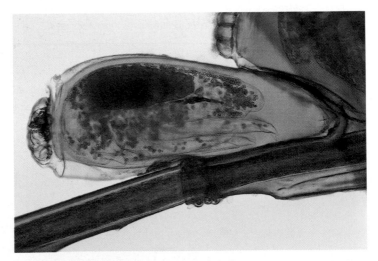

Fig. 5.4 Head louse eggs cemented to a hair shaft.

CLINICAL FEATURES

Itching is the main symptom. Nits tend to be more numerous in the occipital region of the scalp and above the ears. Occasionally, flakes of dandruff or keratin casts may be mistaken for nits, but the distinction is obvious if the material is examined microscopically. Adult lice and nymphs will be found without difficulty in heavier infections (Fig. 5.5). Impetigo may occur as a result of inoculation of staphylococci into the skin during scratching; the term 'nitwit' is derived from the substandard performance of children who had large head louse populations, secondary skin sepsis, and probably also anaemia, and were chronically unwell as a result.

TREATMENT

The insecticides malathion and carbaryl were the mainstay of treatment in the UK for many years. Both are efficient pediculicides and ovicides, and several proprietary preparations are available. Recently, synthetic pyrethroids, which are derived from pyrethrin, a naturally occurring plant insecticide, have been introduced for the treatment of head louse infection. Treatment with any of these preparations should be repeated after 7–10 days, to deal with any louse nymphs emerging from surviving eggs. All family contacts should also be treated.

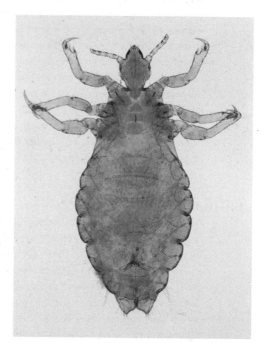

Fig. 5.5 The head louse.

Do not use insecticidal shampoos for the definitive treatment of head louse infection—these expose the insects to a low concentration of insecticide—facilitating the emergence of insecticide resistance in the lice.

INSECTICIDES

- Malathion
- Carbaryl
- Synthetic pyrethroids:
  permethrin
  phenothrin

Body lice (*Pediculus humanus humanus*)

The louse
Has very little 'nous',
Its only pursuit
Is the hirsute.
(I. Kenvyn Evans)

The body, or clothing louse is a parasite of poverty and poor hygiene. It lives, and lays its eggs, on clothing, and only moves onto the body to feed on blood. It is still common in the poorer countries of the world, but in an affluent society its usual hosts are vagrants and down-and-outs who have only one set of clothes which are never removed or cleaned. An individual who regularly changes clothing and maintains a reasonable standard of hygiene will never be a host to body lice, because the lice will not survive laundering and ironing of clothes. Body lice are vectors of epidemic typhus, which has been responsible for millions of deaths over the centuries.

CLINICAL FEATURES

Body lice usually provoke itching, and their host is often covered in excoriations. The itching appears to be the result of an acquired hypersensitivity to louse salivary antigens. Occasionally there is little or no itching, and in these circumstances there may be an enormous number of lice. The sock in Fig. 5.6 belonged to a patient who was teeming with lice, but had no skin lesions of any significance. If you suspect body louse infection there is no point in searching the patient for lice—you should examine the clothing.

Fig. 5.6 Body lice on clothing.

TREATMENT

All the patient requires is a bath. Underclothing should be laundered, and any lice and eggs in the outer-clothing will be killed by 15 minutes in a tumble-dryer.

Crab lice (*Pthirus pubis*)

It's no good standing on the seat
The crabs in here can jump ten feet.
If you think that's rather high,
Go next door, the buggers fly!
      (Toilet graffito)

The crab louse, or pubic louse, in spite of the above allegation of contagion from toilets, is probably most frequently transmitted by direct physical contact with an infected individual. It has always been considered to be rather sedentary, but recent studies suggest that the crab louse becomes animated when its host is sleeping. It is adapted to living in hair of a particular density. It cannot colonize scalp hair, except at the margins of the scalp, but pubic, axillary, beard, and eyelash hair are perfectly acceptable to it, as is the hair on the rest of the body. The crab louse is so named because of its squat shape and powerful claws, resembling a crab's pincers (Fig. 5.7), with which it grasps hair. Female crab lice, like head lice, stick their eggs to hair shafts with a cement material.

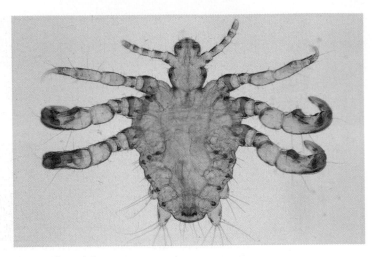

Fig. 5.7 The crab louse.

CLINICAL FEATURES

Itching is the symptom which draws attention to these little passengers. Self-examination usually reveals the reason for the itch, and the patient often presents the doctor with a small envelope, or folded piece of paper, containing specimens. Always open the folded paper carefully, as it has a tendency to flick the crab lice in all directions, leaving one anxiously awaiting signs of personal contamination for weeks thereafter!

Lice are usually visible on the pubic area or in the axillae, but sometimes their eggs, which are brown, are easier to see. If the parasites are very numerous the underclothes may be speckled with spots of altered blood excreted by the lice. Lice on the eyelids festoon the lashes with their eggs (Fig. 5.8).

TREATMENT

Most of the insecticide preparations used in the treatment of head lice may also be used to eradicate crab lice, but alcohol base preparations are irritant on the scrotum, and it is preferable to use an aqueous base preparation such as malathion liquid or lindane lotion. Apply the insecticide from the neck to the toes, and treat the scalp if you see any evidence of lice on the scalp margins. Sexual contacts should also be treated. The treatment should be repeated after an interval of 7–10 days.

Eyelash involvement may also be treated with the aqueous base insecticides, smeared over the lids and lashes, or by application of white soft paraffin several times daily for 2–3 weeks.

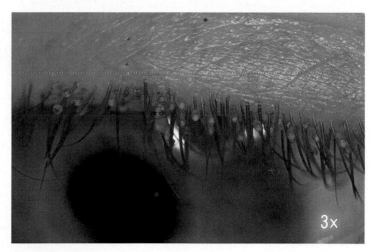

Fig. 5.8 Crab louse eggs on the eyelashes.

PAPULAR URTICARIA

Usually referred to as 'heat bumps' by patients, papular urticaria is a typical response to the bites of a number of arthropods, including biting flies, mosquitoes, mites, fleas and bed-bugs. The lesions are small urticated papules (Fig. 5.9), often surmounted by a tiny vesicle, and they are so itchy that their tops are rapidly excoriated. They arise as a result of a hypersensitivity response to antigens in the arthropods' saliva. Not everyone reacts to these antigens, and in those who do, tolerance is often acquired after a variable length of time.

FLEAS

May the fleas of a thousand camels infest your armpits! (Arab curse)

The commonest cause of papular urticaria acquired in the home environment is flea bites. It is not the human flea, *Pulex irritans*, which is responsible, but fleas whose natural hosts are household pets. A familiar clinical picture is of multiple lesions around the ankles of women (Fig. 5.10). Men are rarely affected, because socks and trousers deny the fleas access to the ankles.

Cats and dogs are perambulating quadripedal 'meals-on-wheels' for the fleas, and although adult fleas can be found on the animals it is really the household which is infested. Flea eggs are not sticky, and when laid by

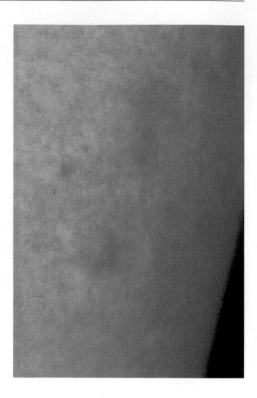

Fig. 5.9 Papular urticaria.

fleas feeding on an animal they drop out of the coat into the surroundings. Flea eggs, larvae, pupae, and adults are present in the carpets and on soft furnishings. Hence, the house should be treated, as well as the pets therein. One of the most effective preparations to deal with flea infestation is a combination of an insecticide, permethrin, with methoprene, a synthetic equivalent of an insect growth regulatory hormone, in an aerosol can (Acclaim Plus). The methoprene blocks the metamorphosis of flea larvae into adults. This should be sprayed on the carpets and soft furnishings, and the animals' sleeping areas, and will confer protection against flea infestation for 4 months. A more recent addition to the anti-flea armamentarium is lufenuron (Program), which is given orally to the animal, is ingested by feeding fleas, and interferes with the production of chitin by flea larvae, thereby preventing their further development.

Occasionally bird fleas will gain access to homes from nests under the eaves, and may be responsible for more extensive lesions of papular urticaria.

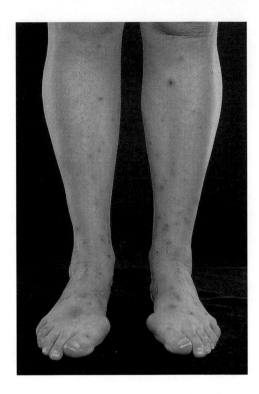

Fig. 5.10 Flea bites on the ankles.

BED-BUGS (*CIMEX LECTULARIUS*)

The butterfly has wings of gold,
The firefly wings of flame,
The bed-bug has no wings at all,
But he gets there just the same.

Bed-bugs are not the most appealing of creatures. They live in dilapidated housing behind peeling wallpaper and rotten skirting boards, and emerge an hour or so before dawn to feed on the sleeping occupants of bedrooms. They feed on blood, and although the process of feeding does not cause the host any pain, a reaction to the bites of the bugs usually results in papular urticaria or bullous lesions. These insects are 5–6 mm long, dark-brown in colour, and can move quite rapidly. Fortunately, bed-bug infestation of houses is now uncommon, but if it is suspected the local Environmental Health Department should be asked to inspect the property.

ANIMAL MITES

Human contact with animals suffering from sarcoptic mange may result in the development of scattered, itchy papules, often on areas coming into contact with the animals—for example, the abdomen and thighs if a mangy dog sits on its owner's lap. It is extremely rare for these animal mites to establish themselves on humans, although there have been a few reported cases.

Dogs, cats and rabbits are the natural hosts of *Cheyletiella* mites, and these may cause skin lesions in humans. Dogs are the usual culprits. On the animal, the mites provoke a heavy scurf over the back ('walking dandruff'), but hardly bother it otherwise. On the owner, itchy papules appear principally on the abdomen, but occasionally also on the thighs and arms—sites of contact with the animal. The diagnosis can be confirmed by taking combings from the animal's coat and demonstrating the mite microscopically. Once the animal has been treated by a veterinary practitioner the human skin lesions resolve spontaneously.

Bird mites may gain access to houses from nests under the eaves, and can cause itchy papular lesions.

TICKS

Ticks are very common, particularly in wooded areas where there are deer populations. They feed on blood, and their barbed mouthparts are held in the skin of the host during feeding by a protein cement material. If a tick is pulled off the skin abruptly, its mouthparts may be left *in situ*, and will provoke a foreign-body reaction.

Ticks are vectors of Lyme disease which is caused by the spirochaete *Borrelia burgdorferi*. Lyme disease (named after the town in Connecticut where its association with ticks was first discovered) affects the skin, joints, central nervous system, and the heart. It responds to treatment with penicillin or tetracyclines.

Probably the best method of tick removal is to grasp it as close to the skin as possible, and exert gentle continuous traction.

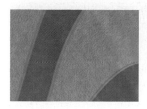

CHAPTER 6

Acne, Acneiform Eruptions and Rosacea

Out, damned spot! Out, I say!
(Shakespeare, *Macbeth* v.i)

INTRODUCTION

This chapter deals with disorders which give rise to papules and pustules, often known in the vernacular as 'spots' or 'zits'. Some are aetiologically related and can properly be called variants of acne (a corruption of the Greek *akme*—a point). Others produce lesions closely or superficially resembling 'true' acne: the acneiform disorders and rosacea. A summary of the acne family is as follows:

THE ACNE FAMILY

Acne vulgaris
- 'Classical'
- Infantile and juvenile onset
- Late-onset
- Severe (acne conglobata; nodulocystic)
- With systemic symptoms (acne fulminans)

Secondary acne
- Endocrine-associated

Continued on p. 72

71

THE ACNE FAMILY *(Continued)*

- Medicaments
- Oils
- Chloracne

Hidradenitis suppurativa

ACNE VULGARIS AND ITS VARIANTS

Acne vulgaris

About 80% of people develop some spottiness. Acne may be very mild indeed but at its most severe, gross and unsightly changes are seen.

Acne may be associated with underlying endocrinological abnormalities (see below) but usually it is not.

AGE OF ONSET AND COURSE

The first problems are usually encountered in adolescence, although there are exceptions (see below).

Lesions of acne vary considerably with time. Most patients notice marked fluctuations in the number and severity of the spots. In girls, this is often related to the menstrual cycle. The condition frequently deteriorates at times of stress.

Overall severity tends to increase initially before gradually settling after 2–3 years, and disappearing altogether in the majority. The peak of severity is earlier in girls than boys. In some individuals the time-course may be much more prolonged, lesions continuing to develop well into adult life.

There are two groups in whom true acne develops outside adolescence.

Infantile/juvenile acne

Typical acne is occasionally seen in infants and children (especially boys), usually at 3–12 months of age. Although lesions subside after 4–5 years, adolescence often heralds a severe recrudescence. Endocrine abnormalities are very rarely found, but should be considered, especially in a girl with signs of virilism.

Late-onset acne

Some women develop acne in their thirties and forties, often with marked pre-menstrual exacerbations. Endocrinological investigation is generally unrewarding, but some have polycystic ovary syndrome (see p. 82).

THE PSYCHOLOGICAL IMPACT OF ACNE

Acne can make life really miserable. Its predilection for the teens and twenties means that acne affects those who are least well-equipped to cope.

The face is prominently involved, and in adolescence the face assumes increasing importance as part of an attractive image. At the time when acne strikes, the individual is also moving towards major relationships outside the family and the close circle of same-sex friends: pair-bonding is the new game and it is now that acne wreaks its havoc.

Realize, too, that the psychological impact of acne is not necessarily related to the degree of severity as perceived by an outsider. A young person may spend just as long staring miserably into the mirror when there are only a few spots as when there are hundreds.

CLINICAL FEATURES

Physical signs

The characteristic distribution is as follows.

SITE AND DISTRIBUTION

- Face, any part of which may be involved
- Neck, especially posteriorly
- Upper back
- Anterior chest, in an inverted 'V' from the shoulders to the xiphisternum
- Shoulders
- Ears

In severe acne, lesions may extend down the arms, and the whole of the central back may be affected, with lesions extending on to the buttocks.

The appearance of the skin

The first physical sign to note is that the face and upper trunk become very greasy (Fig. 6.1) due to increased production of sebum. This is normal at puberty, but is excessive in those with bad acne. Scalp hair is often very greasy too. Greasiness alone may be bad enough for the patient to seek advice.

The individual lesions of acne

A cardinal feature is that acne is a polymorphic disorder. There are several different types of lesion at any one time.

ACNE VULGARIS LESIONS

- Comedones:
    closed ('whiteheads')
    open ('blackheads')
- Papules
- Pustules
- Nodules
- Cysts
- Scars

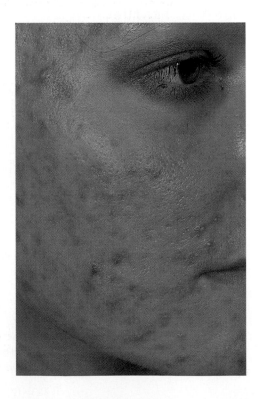

Fig. 6.1 This girl's face shows the typical greasy skin of the acne sufferer, in addition to papules and pustules.

Comedones (singular: comedo)

The presence of comedones is an important diagnostic aid. There are two types: closed (or 'whitehead') and open (or 'blackhead').

Closed comedones are more easily felt than seen. They are very small papules, with a central point or elevation (Fig. 6.2). They are often most numerous on the forehead and cheeks. There is little or no inflammation.

Open comedones (blackheads) are dilated, blocked hair follicles, but it is not entirely clear what causes the characteristic black dots. Burnt-out inflammatory lesions may leave multiheaded blackheads, particularly on the shoulders and upper trunk. Blackheads are virtually pathognomonic of acne in the younger patient (although advanced solar damage may also result in blackhead formation).

Papules and pustules

The majority of patients with acne develop papules and pustules; some have hundreds. They are the well-known little red spots or pustules on a red base. They may itch or be quite painful. Papules develop rapidly, often over a few hours, and frequently become pustular as they evolve. They resolve over the course of a few days. New lesions may arise in exactly the same site on many occasions.

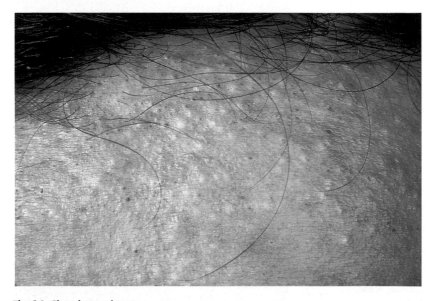

Fig. 6.2 Closed comedones.

Nodules and cysts

With increasing severity, and as the inflammation extends deeper, the size of visible and palpable lesions increases, resulting in deep-seated nodules and cysts (Fig. 6.3). Many patients develop a few, but some have large numbers, and this is the situation in which the term 'acne conglobata' is used.

These severe lesions are often extremely uncomfortable and last much longer than more superficial changes. Some become chronic, and may result in permanent cyst formation (see Chapter 9).

Scars

The final common pathway for the inflammatory process of acne is scarring, which will remain as a lifetime's legacy of adolescent anguish. Charac-

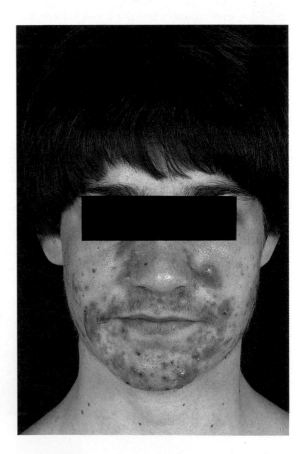

Fig. 6.3 Acne conglobata.

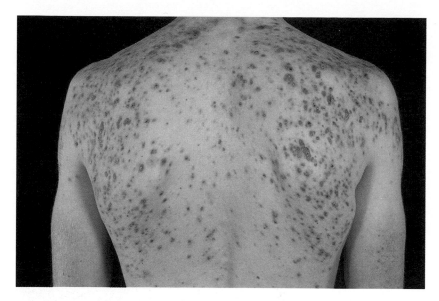

Fig. 6.3 Continued.

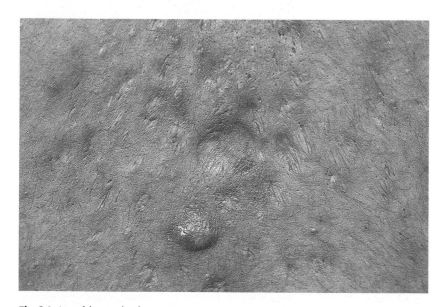

Fig. 6.4 Atrophic scarring in acne.

teristically, small, deep 'ice-pick' scars occur, but more severe disease can leave gross changes, with atrophy (Fig. 6.4) or keloid formation (see Chapter 9).

Systemic symptoms (acne fulminans)

Very occasionally a young man with severe nodulocystic acne develops fever, malaise and joint pain and swelling. This is known as 'acne fulminans'.

PATHOGENESIS OF ACNE

The aetio-pathology of acne remains to be elucidated fully. However, it seems that several key features contribute to the final picture (see Fig. 6.5), but it should be noted that this does not fully explain every aspect of the disorder, for example the occurrence of pre-pubertal acne.

As the inflammation subsides, a variable amount of fibrosis occurs. This may produce scarring, particularly if repeated episodes occur in the same site. Sometimes epithelial remnants become walled-off by fibrosis, producing cysts.

PATHOGENESIS OF ACNE

1 Androgens (usually in normal amounts) stimulate increased sebum production
2 Hair follicles with particularly large sebaceous glands (on the face, neck, chest and back) become blocked by hyperkeratosis
3 This results in the closed comedo
4 Within the follicle, an obligate anaerobe (*Propionibacterium acnes*) proliferates
5 This organism acts on sebum, releasing inflammatory chemicals
6 These leak into the surrounding dermis
7 The body mounts an intense acute inflammatory response

The result of this is the papule, pustule or nodule

TREATMENT OF ACNE

Treatments available for the management of acne.

Topical therapies

Benzoyl peroxide is widely used because it reduces comedones (it is 'comedolytic'). It must be used regularly and in the long term. There are several strengths, and it is best to start with a weak preparation, applied once daily, and gradually progress to stronger preparations.

THE PATHOGENESIS OF ACNE

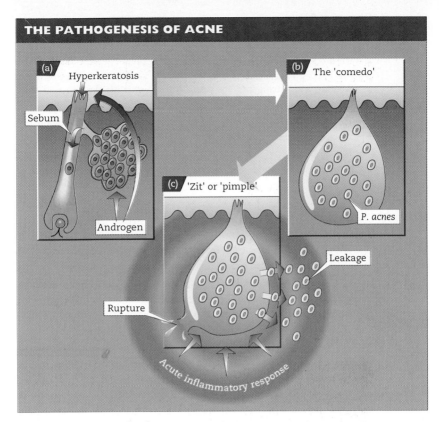

Fig. 6.5 The pathogenesis of acne.

TREATMENTS

Topical
- Benzoyl peroxide
- Retinoic acid
- Sulphur and astringents
- Topical antiseptics
- Topical antibiotics

Systemic
- Antibiotics
- Cyproterone acetate
- 13-cis retinoic acid (isotretinoin)
- Steroids

Surgical intervention

Retinoic acid is a derivative of vitamin A, and also has comedolytic activity.

Sulphur and astringents are preparations which make the skin flaky and thereby unblock hair follicles.

Topical antiseptics such as povidone iodine and chlorhexidine are often prescribed, but are of little proven value.

Topical tetracyclines, erythromycin and clindamycin are available, and are generally applied once daily. All have been shown to be useful in milder acne.

Systemic therapies

Antibiotics are the mainstay of the treatment of papulopustular acne. It is not known precisely how they work, but they reduce bacterial counts, at least initially, and may also have direct anti-inflammatory effects.

The most effective are the tetracyclines and erythromycin. To work, antibiotics must be fat soluble, and the *penicillins are therefore useless.* Most tetracyclines should be taken on an empty stomach. Tetracyclines are contraindicated in the under-12s, and in pregnancy and lactation.

Cyproterone acetate is an antiandrogen which can only be given to women. It is given with oestrogen to prevent menorrhagia and to ensure contraceptive cover (it will feminize a male fetus). Its effect is rather slow.

13-*cis* retinoic acid (isotretinoin) is a highly effective oral vitamin A derivative which dramatically reduces sebum production. It has several side-effects: dry lips, eyes and skin, nose-bleeds, mild alopecia, aches and pains. It also raises blood fat levels and may affect liver function tests. The most serious problem is teratogenicity. *Female patients must not become pregnant when taking isotretinoin, as it will produce fetal abnormalities.* Isotretinoin is only available on hospital prescription in the UK.

Over 90% of patients have complete clearance of their acne and in most there is no relapse.

Steroids can be used intralesionally or systemically in severe acne (they are virtually always needed in acne fulminans).

Surgical intervention

Simple measures, such as removing multiple comedones with a comedone extractor may improve the appearance. It certainly gives great pleasure and satisfaction to girl- or boy-friend who likes to pop out blackheads! Large, residual cysts may need to be excised, but there is a risk of keloid scarring. Plastic surgeons can sometimes help acne scarring by dermabrasion, but this must not be attempted until the acne is fully under control.

MANAGEMENT OF A PATIENT WITH ACNE

The approach to treatment must be tailored to the individual, but there are some general guidelines which may be helpful. Let's first dispel some myths!

COMMON ACNE MYTHS

- Acne is due to fatty food or sweets
- Acne is due to being dirty
- Acne is due to 'hormonal imbalance'
- Acne is related to sexual behaviour

All rubbish!

- Diet plays no role at all; there is no need to avoid sweets, chocolate or chips
- Even hourly washing would make no difference
- Hormones are normal in the vast majority
- Neither too little, nor too much sex makes any difference (thank goodness!)

Assessment of the patient

It can be useful to consider acne in three broad severity bands: mild, moderate and severe.

Mild acne may respond to topical treatment alone. Begin with benzoyl peroxide or retinoic acid, and possibly try a topical antibiotic.

Moderate acne should initially be treated with a combination of benzoyl peroxide and oral tetracycline, oxytetracycline or erythromycin

ACNE ASSESSMENT

Mild
Only comedones *and/or*
only a few papulopustular lesions
restricted to the face

Moderate
More papulopustular lesions on the
face or over a wider area *and/or*
occasional nodules

Severe
Very widespread papulopustular
lesions *and/or*
nodulocystic lesions *and/or*
systemic symptoms
or
acne of moderate severity, failing to
settle within 6 months of therapy
or
acne of whatever severity with
significant psychological upset

in a dose of 500 mg twice daily. Continue for at least 3–6 months before reassessing. Alternative tetracyclines have their advocates: some may be better absorbed or tolerated, but most are more expensive and there is generally no indication for their use as first-line agents.

If the response is not satisfactory, the acne should be managed as outlined below.

Severe acne may be controlled to some extent by systemic antibiotics, but this degree of acne often demands more aggressive treatment. Girls may respond to cyproterone acetate with or without antibiotics, allowing at least 6 months for a response. Many girls and most young men eventually require 13-*cis* retinoic acid, usually for 4–6 months at a daily dose of 1 mg/kg.

Intralesional steroids are useful for acute inflammatory lesions. Very rarely, systemic steroid therapy may be required, especially in acne fulminans.

Surgical intervention may be required later to help overcome the devastation wreaked by this degree of acne.

SECONDARY ACNE

Acne lesions may arise as a consequence of other primary pathological processes. Such 'secondary' acne is often monomorphic and generally mild.

An exception is acne occurring in patients with *endocrine abnormalities*. The commonest is polycystic ovary syndrome, in which acne of any severity may accompany hirsutism and menstrual irregularities. Any cause of abnormally high circulating androgen levels (such as tumours) may also cause quite severe acne. Milder lesions are seen in Cushing's syndrome.

Medicaments such as greasy ointments, pomades and topical steroids may induce comedones, particularly on the forehead and cheeks. Occasionally, papules may develop. Several drugs induce acneiform lesions or make pre-existing acne worse, e.g. systemic steroids, phenytoin, isoniazid and lithium.

Oil-induced acne occurs when mineral oils come into close contact with the skin. This is often at unusual sites, such as the lower abdomen and thighs.

Chloracne is a specific change in which comedones appear after exposure to chlorinated chemical compounds. A famous example was the release of dioxin from the explosion at Seveso in Italy. Systemic upsets also occur.

HIDRADENITIS SUPPURATIVA

Although uncommon, this distinctive disorder results in very unpleasant chronic, relapsing sepsis in the apocrine glands of the axillae and groins (Fig. 6.6). Lesions may appear on the breasts (which are modified apocrine glands).

Recurrent painful abscesses and sinus tracks develop. Many patients with hidradenitis have concurrent severe acne, or have suffered from acne in the past.

Some patients improve on long-term antibiotics, but many require plastic surgery.

ACNEIFORM DISORDERS

Several conditions mimic acne. In most, close examination will reveal important differences.

Pseudofolliculitis barbae (shaving rash): produces small papules in the beard area and is commoner in those with naturally curly hair, especially

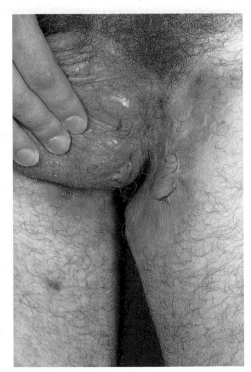

Fig. 6.6 Hidradenitis suppurativa.

Afro-Caribbeans. Occasionally small keloids develop. The process may involve the nape of the neck, when it is usually termed *acne keloidalis*. Treatment is unsatisfactory.

Acne excoriée (des jeunes filles) is typically seen in teenage girls who present with facial excoriations. Examination reveals very few primary lesions, and there are no comedones. This is not true acne but a form of neurotic excoriation (see Chapter 20). Tranquillizers may help.

Pityrosporum folliculitis causes follicular papules and pustules on the trunk, without other features of acne. The condition responds to antifungal agents such as miconazole.

Keratosis pilaris is the name given to small spiky projections at the mouth of hair follicles, most often seen on the upper, outer arms and shoulders (Fig. 6.7). However, lesions may appear on the face, especially in children, and are occasionally pustular. A family history is common. Topical retinoic acid may be helpful.

Fig. 6.7 Keratosis pilaris on the upper arm.

Rosacea is an important differential diagnosis of acne, and is sometimes called 'acne rosacea'. It most frequently affects middle-aged women, but it may occur in men, and can occur much earlier in life. The sites of predilection are the central cheeks, forehead and glabellar region, end of the nose and chin (Fig. 6.8). The eruption consists of small papules and pustules arising in crops on an erythematous, telangiectatic background.

There are no comedones. Patients frequently complain that their face flushes easily with heat or alcohol, and migraines are more common. In men, severe involvement of the nose leads to marked sebaceous hyperplasia known as *rhinophyma* (Fig. 6.9).

The treatment of choice is tetracyclines, given for several weeks in similar doses to those for moderate acne (see above). Topical metronidazole or sulphur/salicylic acid creams may help. It may be possible to tail off the treatment, but the condition often recurs. Topical steroids make matters worse.

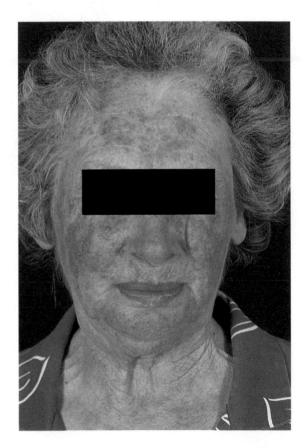

Fig. 6.8 Typical rosacea.

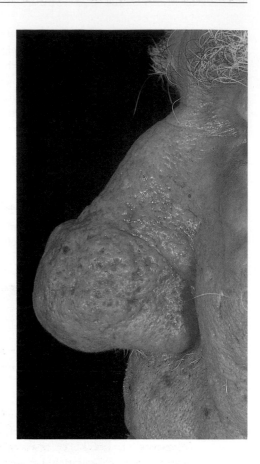

Fig. 6.9 Rhinophyma.

Perioral dermatitis (note for strict classical scholars: it should really be 'circum-oral') produces a clinical appearance somewhat reminiscent of rosacea (see Fig. 22.2), and is often associated with topical steroid abuse. (For more details see Chapter 22.)

CHAPTER 7

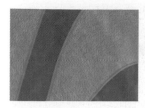

Eczema

To keep three or four spots of eczema in a private part of my body and now and then to scald or bathe them with hot water behind closed doors. Ah, is this not happiness? (Tim Shangt'an)

The terms eczema (Greek, meaning 'to boil over') and dermatitis are synonymous. They are applied to a particular type of inflammatory reaction pattern in the skin which may be provoked by a number of external or internal factors.

CLINICAL FEATURES

The principal symptom of eczema is itching. The clinical signs depend on its aetiology, site, and duration, but usually comprise erythema, oedema, papules, vesicles, and exudation (Fig. 7.1). An acute eczema will have all these features, and may also have a bullous component. In a chronic eczema oedema is not a prominent feature, but the epidermis becomes thickened and the skin surface markings are exaggerated (lichenification) (Fig. 7.2). A common feature of chronic eczema of the hands and feet is the formation of painful fissures in the skin overlying joints.

A phenomenon which is seen particularly with an acute dermatitis is secondary spread of the eczema to sites distant from the originally affected area. In some cases this response is triggered by an external allergen, but in others there is no obvious explanation for it. Occasionally, most of the body surface is affected, and eczema is one cause of generalized exfoliative dermatitis.

Other changes in the skin which may accompany eczema include scratch marks and secondary bacterial infection. Prolonged scratching and

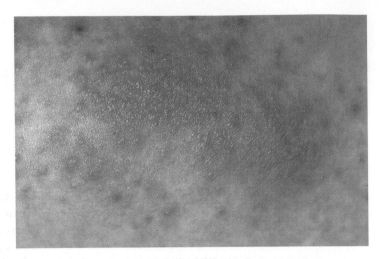

Fig. 7.1 Typical eczema.

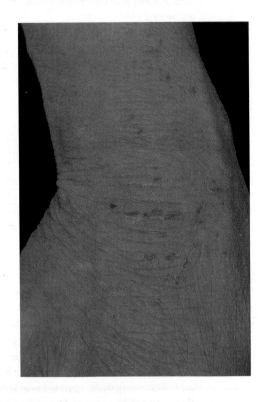

Fig. 7.2 Lichenified eczema.

rubbing of the skin tends to polish the finger-nails, which may look very shiny.

CLASSIFICATION

We still have a great deal to learn about the aetiology of certain types of eczema, so any attempt at classification is based upon our present state of ignorance. The most frequently employed system of classification divides cases of eczema into 'exogenous' where an external agent is responsible, and 'endogenous' where the problem is principally constitutional. There are, however, frequent cases in which more than one factor may be operating—for example, the hairdresser with hand dermatitis who suffers from atopic eczema and also has a superimposed irritant dermatitis from shampoos. Do not be too rigid in your attempts to classify a particular dermatitis—it may not fit a recognized category and you may find yourself using more general terms such as 'probably endogenous'. The following classification includes most of the types of eczema you are likely to encounter.

ECZEMA CLASSIFICATION

Exogenous
- Primary irritant dermatitis
- Allergic contact dermatitis

Endogenous
- Atopic eczema
- Seborrhoeic dermatitis
- Discoid eczema
- Varicose eczema
- Endogenous eczema of palms and soles
- Asteatotic eczema

Exogenous eczema

PRIMARY IRRITANT DERMATITIS

Primary irritants physically damage the skin; they include acids, alkalis, detergents, and petroleum products. Some strong irritants will produce an immediate effect, whereas with weaker irritants the effects are cumulative. Anyone suffering from constitutional eczema is more susceptible to the effects of primary irritants. The person who does a lot of housework is a good candidate for a cumulative primary irritant dermatitis, because his/

her hands will be perpetually immersed in washing-up liquid, dirty nappies and soap-powder.

Occupational irritant dermatitis is common. During the early part of their training, hairdressing apprentices spend a substantial part of the day with their hands immersed in shampoo on their clients' heads, and many develop irritant dermatitis. If they also have a constitutional eczema, such as atopic eczema, their hand problem usually becomes so severe that they are forced to leave hairdressing (Fig. 7.3). A similar situation is seen in machine-tool operators whose hands are immersed in cutting fluids.

In theory, the treatment is simple—either remove the patient from contact with the irritant, or protect the hands against it. This may be feasible in some occupations, but in others it is not. With present employment problems most people are reluctant to give up their jobs, and many are unable to wear gloves at work. The skin can be helped to a certain extent by the liberal use of emollients (see Chapter 22), but it cannot be restored to normal whilst exposure to irritants continues. What usually happens is that severe dermatitis eventually forces a change of occupation, or individuals with milder problems learn to tolerate them.

ALLERGIC CONTACT DERMATITIS

This is due to a delayed hypersensitivity reaction to an external allergen. There are innumerable chemicals which can act as allergens, but most rarely cause problems. Some chemicals are such potent allergens that they will sensitize after one exposure, but many require multiple exposures

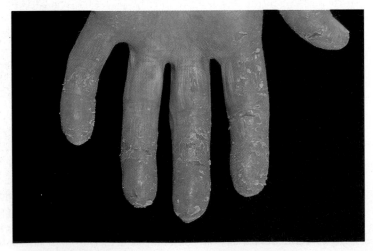

Fig. 7.3 Severe dermatitis of the hands in a hairdresser.

before sensitization occurs. It is possible to be exposed to an allergen for years, and then suddenly develop hypersensitivity.

Frequent causes of contact dermatitis include nickel, colophony, rubber additives, chromate, hair dyes, and topical medicaments—both their active ingredients and components of their bases.

Nickel dermatitis

Nickel is the commonest cause of contact dermatitis in women. Sensitization usually occurs as a result of wearing inexpensive costume jewellery. The problem usually begins with sore, itchy ear-lobes, but it is dermatitis caused by other metallic components of garments which brings the nickel-sensitive patient to the dermatologist. In the pre-mini-skirt era, suspender dermatitis was the commonest presentation of nickel sensitivity. The metal clips produced patches of dermatitis on the thighs. With the advent of the mini-skirt and tights, suspender dermatitis became a thing of the past. The clips and hooks on modern underwear are coated metal or synthetic material, and rarely cause problems. It is the jeans stud which has become one of the principal sources of nickel on the modern person. A patch of eczema adjacent to the umbilicus is virtually pathognomonic of nickel sensitivity (Fig. 7.4).

If nickel dermatitis is suspected, look at the skin on the ear-lobes, and under the wrist-watch. Many people who are aware that inexpensive

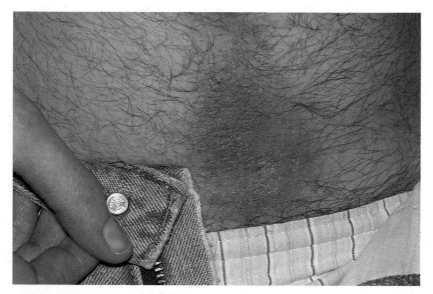

Fig. 7.4 Contact dermatitis to nickel in jeans stud.

earrings provoke a reaction will continue to wear them from time to time. Nickel dermatitis on the wrists is usually caused by the metal buckle on a watch-strap, but may also be due to bracelets. Stainless steel does not appear to cause any problems, because although steel contains nickel it does not leach out.

Anyone who is nickel sensitive should be advised to avoid costume jewellery, bare metal clips on underwear, metal buckles on shoes, and metal zips. The metal stud on the front of jeans can be replaced by a button, and problems from watches can usually be avoided by wearing a 'Swatch' watch, as the only metal in contact with the skin is the stainless steel battery compartment.

Colophony

This is a resin which is a component of some adhesive plasters.

Rubber dermatitis

The rubber we encounter in day-to-day life contains numerous chemicals which can cause contact dermatitis. They are used to speed up the vulcanization of rubber (accelerators) and to prevent its oxidation (antioxidants). Rubber glove dermatitis used to be common, but is less frequent now. The commonest presentation of rubber contact dermatitis is shoe dermatitis—provoked by rubber components and rubber adhesives in shoes.

Chromate

Chromium compounds have a number of industrial applications. They are also used in leather tanning, and are the major sensitizer in cement. Cement dermatitis is common in building workers.

Hair dye dermatitis

Contact sensitivity to hair dye usually presents as a severe dermatitis affecting the ears, face and eyelids. Hair dyes are also a frequent cause of allergic contact dermatitis on the hands in hairdressers.

Topical medicaments

Medicament dermatitis is quite common in dermatological practice, but relatively infrequent if one considers the huge quantities of creams, lotions and potions used in an average household. Common causes include antibiotics, particularly neomycin, local anaesthetics (except lignocaine, which is a rare sensitizer), antihistamines, preservatives such as parabens and ethylenediamine, and lanolin. Dermatoses in which medicament contact sensitivity may be a complicating factor include otitis externa, pruritus ani and varicose ulcers.

Occupational contact dermatitis

A detailed history about the nature of a patient's work is absolutely essential. A history of improvement during holiday periods is typical of a work-related dermatosis. Ask the patient precisely what their job entails—it is common to encounter terminology which is specific to a certain occupation, and is incomprehensible to those outside the trade. Establish what materials are handled at work, and if there have been any changes which coincided with the onset of the dermatitis. Do any workmates have similar problems? It is sometimes necessary to see a patient in his/her working environment.

Plant dermatitis

Plant dermatitis is relatively uncommon in the UK, but the Primulae, particularly *Primula obconica*, are the plants usually responsible. In the USA the commonest cause of plant dermatitis is poison ivy. Dermatitis caused by plants tends to present with a linear, vesiculobullous reaction on the exposed parts of the body (see Fig. 15.12).

Diagnosis of allergic contact dermatitis

It is important to take a detailed history covering present occupation, previous occupations, hobbies, and the use of topical medicaments. The distribution pattern of the dermatitis may suggest a possible allergen, and provoke further questions—for example, eczema adjacent to the umbilicus prompts questions about previous problems with earrings. Certain patterns are characteristic of a particular allergen: eczema on the face, in the ears, on the hands, and on one or other thigh is typical of contact sensitivity to phosphorus sesquisulphide in 'strike anywhere' matches. The facial eczema is caused by particles of this chemical in the smoke from the matches; the hand eczema by handling the box, which has the chemical on the striking surface; that on the thigh from carrying the box in the pocket; and that in the ears from using matches to clean them out!

However, when the cause is not as obvious it may require considerable detective work to track it down.

Patch testing (see Chapter 2) is of considerable help in the investigation of allergic contact dermatitis. This procedure is quite different from prick or scratch testing. It is a delayed hypersensitivity response, in which the reaction takes 48 hours to develop, whereas prick or scratch tests elicit an immediate hypersensitivity response which develops within minutes. A standard battery of common allergens is used in routine patch testing, but other batteries of allergens encountered in particular occupations are also available. The majority of the allergens used are mixed in white soft paraffin to a specific concentration—many allergens are irritant in high concentration and will produce false-positive reactions. Patients may claim they are 'allergic' to materials they use at work, and these are usually presented to the dermatologist in unmarked jars. Such materials are often irritants, and if used undiluted for patch testing may bore a large, untidy hole in the patient's back.

Positive patch test reactions must be interpreted in the context of the patient's presenting problem—not all positives will be relevant.

Wait until an acute eczema has settled before patch testing—positive reactions may exacerbate the eczema.

Treatment

Potent topical steroids (see Chapter 22) should be used to settle the eczema prior to patch testing. Once an allergen has been identified as the cause of a problem, the patient should be advised about its avoidance. If components of medicaments are involved, the patient's general practitioner must be informed of what preparations the patient should avoid.

Endogenous eczema

ATOPIC ECZEMA

'Atopy' implies a genetic predisposition to develop eczema, asthma and hay fever. A family history of atopy is common in patients with atopic eczema. The pathogenesis of atopic eczema is complex, and other factors, such as environmental influences and emotional stimuli, may play a role.

Atopic eczema is not present at birth, but frequently appears in the first year of life. In early childhood the eczema is often generalized, but later a characteristic flexural involvement is seen—wrists, antecubital fossae, popliteal fossae, and dorsa of feet (Fig. 7.5). The skin is dry and intensely itchy. As a result of constant scratching and rubbing, the affected areas become thickened (lichenification). The course is typically punctuated by episodic exacerbations.

Atopic eczema often resolves in childhood, but may persist into adolescence and adult life, and there is no way of predicting the outcome. Those whose eczema has cleared remain susceptible to the effects of primary irritants, and should avoid occupations such as hairdressing and engineering.

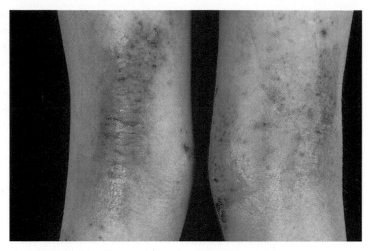

Fig. 7.5 Flexural involvement in atopic eczema.

The commonest complication is secondary bacterial infection, producing folliculitis or impetigo. Viral warts and molluscum contagiosum occur more frequently in atopics, and herpes simplex infection may lead to widespread skin lesions (see Chapter 3) and a severe illness (eczema herpeticum; Kaposi's varicelliform eruption).

Treatment

An important aspect of the management of a child with atopic eczema is sympathetic explanation of the nature of the condition to its parents.

Emollients are essential in the management of the dry skin in atopic eczema. There are numerous emollients available, and it may be necessary to change preparations to find which are most suitable for a particular individual. They can be used in combination at bathtime—for example, one as a soap substitute, a bath oil in the water, and an emollient cream afterwards.

Topical steroids are invaluable in the treatment of atopic eczema. In young children mild, non-fluorinated steroids such as hydrocortisone are the mainstay. In older children and adults more potent steroids are required, but the aim should always be to use the weakest preparation sufficient to control the disease. A topical steroid/antibacterial combination may be useful if eczema frequently becomes secondarily infected—obvious secondary infection should be treated with a systemic antibiotic such as flucloxacillin or erythromycin.

Medicated bandages such as zinc paste and ichthammd or zinc oxide and coal tar, applied over a topical steroid, are useful in the management of severe eczema on the limbs. A sedative antihistamine at night may help to reduce scratching. Ultraviolet light treatment, either UVB or psoralens and ultraviolet A (therapy), (PUVA), helps some atopics, but the eczema often relapses when treatment is stopped.

The influence of diet on atopic eczema is contentious. In some children, replacement of cows' milk by a soya preparation results in some improvement, but in the majority it does not appear to help. Most dermatologists reserve dietary manipulation for severely affected children who fail to benefit from other treatment methods. It is dangerous to manipulate a child's diet without expert advice, as this can lead to nutritional deficiencies.

SEBORRHOEIC DERMATITIS

This is a constitutional disorder whose exact pathogenesis is not fully understood, but recently the role of *Pityrosporum* yeasts has been emphasized.

Seborrhoeic dermatitis affects the scalp, face, pre-sternal area, upper back, and flexures. Scalp involvement presents as itchy, diffuse scaling on an erythematous background. On the face, there is scaly erythema in the naso-labial folds and on the forehead, eyebrows, and beard area (Fig. 7.6).

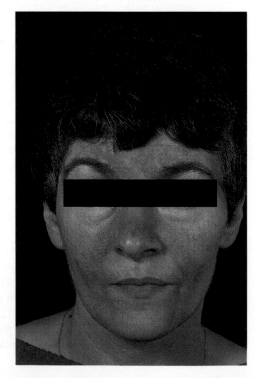

Fig. 7.6 Facial seborrhoeic dermatitis.

Lesions on the chest are often marginated. Flexural involvement produces a moist, glazed erythema.

Seborrhoeic dermatitis usually responds to topical hydrocortisone, but will recur when treatment is stopped. It is important to explain this to the patient, who will otherwise be tempted to try more potent topical steroids in an attempt to find a 'cure'. Tar shampoos and steroid lotions or gels will help the scalp. The apparent involvement of *Pityrosporum* has prompted the use of topical ketoconazole cream and shampoo, both of which appear to be beneficial.

DISCOID ECZEMA

In this disorder, scattered, well-demarcated areas of eczema develop on the trunk and limbs. A potent topical steroid is usually required to keep the condition controlled. Its aetiology is unknown.

VARICOSE ECZEMA

Chronic venous hypertension is frequently associated with eczematous changes on the legs. Secondary spread to the forearms is common.

Mild or moderate potency topical steroids will usually suppress the eczema.

ENDOGENOUS ECZEMA OF THE PALMS AND SOLES

Some patients develop symmetrical chronic eczema on the palms and soles, unrelated to external factors. Long-term treatment with potent topical steroids is usually required.

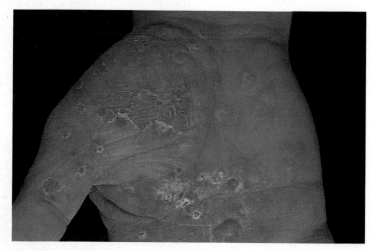

Fig. 7.7 Pompholyx.

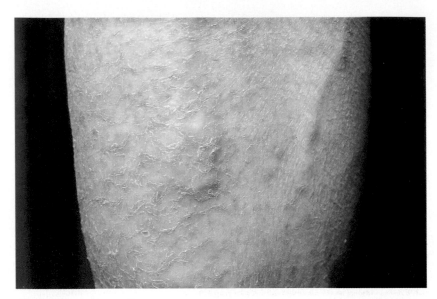

Fig. 7.8 Eczema craquelé.

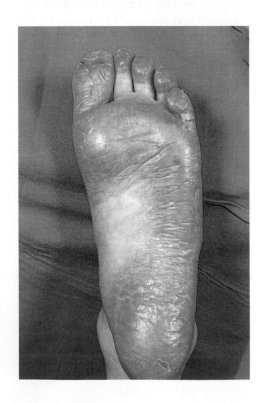

Fig. 7.9 Juvenile plantar dermatosis.

An episodic form of eczema of the palms and soles, in which bulla formation occurs, is known as *acute pompholyx* (Fig. 7.7).This develops rapidly, and can be severely incapacitating. Secondary bacterial infection is common. It usually responds to treatment with potassium permanganate soaks and a systemic antibiotic.The trigger for these episodes is unknown.

ASTEATOTIC ECZEMA (ECZEMA CRAQUELÉ)

With increasing age, the lipid content of the stratum corneum decreases, and elderly skin is particularly susceptible to 'degreasing' agents. Asteatotic eczema is usually seen on the legs, but may also occur on the lower abdomen and arms, and occasionally it is generalized. It is common in elderly patients admitted to hospital and bathed more frequently than they bathe at home. A crazy-paving pattern develops (Fig. 7.8), and the skin begins to itch.Treatment with an emollient is usually suffcient, but a more troublesome exudative eczema may develop, and this requires topical steroid therapy.

JUVENILE PLANTAR DERMATOSIS

As its name suggests, this condition occurs in children. It is thought to be related to wearing socks made of synthetic materials and training shoes. The weight-bearing areas of the feet are dry and shiny, and painful fissures occur (Fig. 7.9). Changing to cotton or woollen socks and leather shoes sometimes helps, as does the liberal use of emollients.Topical steroids are usually ineffective. It almost invariably resolves by the early teens.

CHAPTER 8

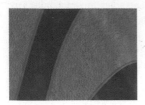

Psoriasis

Dermatologists do it on a grand scale. (Anon)

INTRODUCTION

Psoriasis is one of the commonest and most important of the inflammatory dermatoses: about 1.5% of the population of western countries develop psoriasis during their lifetime. It is also common in India, the Far East, and parts of Africa. As most of those who develop psoriasis have lesions for the rest of their lives, it is clearly a considerable problem.

It is still not known why psoriasis develops. There is a strong genetic component in some people, particularly if the disease begins in youth or early adulthood. However, although a family history is common, there is often no clear-cut inheritance pattern and the 'genetic' explanation may not be readily understood by patients.

Some well-recognized triggers may induce psoriasis in susceptible individuals, notably trauma and infections. Some authorities also maintain that stress may induce or exacerbate the condition. However, there is no clear understanding of what causes some areas of skin to turn into plaques of psoriasis while others remain essentially normal.

PATHOLOGY

The pathological process is a combination of epidermal hyperproliferation and accumulation of inflammatory cells. The 'epidermal transit time' is markedly reduced from the normal 30 days to around 6 days. There is also increased vascularity of the upper dermis. Figure 8.1 shows a schematic representation of a psoriatic plaque. The cardinal features are as follows:

CARDINAL FEATURES

- Marked thickening of the epidermis (acanthosis)
- Absence of the granular cell layer
- Retention of nuclei in the horny layer (parakeratosis)
- Accumulations of polymorphs in the horny layer (microabscesses)
- Dilated capillary loops in the upper dermis

This basic picture, with some variations (e.g. increased size and number of polymorph abscesses in pustular psoriasis), unites all forms of psoriasis. It is also seen in the skin lesions of Reiter's syndrome (see p. 116).

PSORIATIC PLAQUE

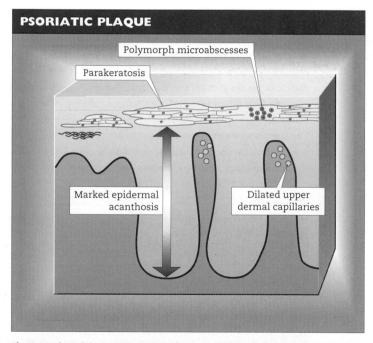

Polymorph microabscesses

Parakeratosis

Marked epidermal acanthosis

Dilated upper dermal capillaries

Fig. 8.1 Schematic representation of a psoriatic plaque.

CLINICAL PATTERNS OF PSORIASIS

A number of different clinical patterns of psoriasis are recognized.

CLINICAL PATTERNS

- Classical plaque
- Scalp psoriasis
- Nail psoriasis
- Guttate
- Flexural
- 'Brittle'
- Erythrodermic
- Acute pustular
- Chronic palmo-plantar pustulosis
- Arthropathic psoriasis

Some are common and others are rarer. Some may be seen together or overlapping with each other. However, there is some merit in considering them separately.

CLASSICAL PLAQUE PSORIASIS

This is the commonest pattern. There are single or multiple plaques, varying from a few millimetres to several centimetres in diameter. The plaques are red and the surface is scaly (Fig. 8.2). If scraped very gently, the scale can be seen to reflect the light, giving a 'silvery' effect (due to the parakeratotic horny layer). More vigorous rubbing induces capillary-point haemorrhage.

The plaques may develop on any part of the body, but psoriasis has a predilection for extensor surfaces: the knees, the elbows and the base of the spine (Fig. 8.2). Lesions are often strikingly symmetrical. Involvement of

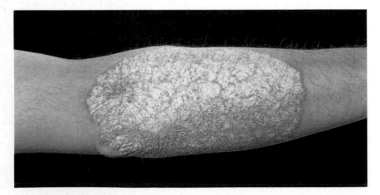

Fig. 8.2 Psoriatic plaque on the elbow.

the face is relatively uncommon. The scalp and nails are often affected (see Figs 8.3–8.4), and an arthropathy may also occur (see p. 114).

Plaques tend to be chronic and stable, with little day-to-day change (as compared with 'brittle' psoriasis—see below). However, they may enlarge slowly, and may merge with adjacent areas. They may also resolve spontaneously. Occasionally, psoriatic plaques appear at the site of trauma or scarring. This is known as the Köbner or isomorphic phenomenon and is a characteristic, but not pathognomonic, feature. Exposure to UV radiation and natural sunlight often (but not always) improve psoriasis.

It is often said that psoriasis is not itchy, but in our experience a significant number of patients complain of severe itching, and most experience some itch at times. In fact the Greek *psora* actually means itch. Some forms of psoriasis (e.g. guttate, flexural) are more prone to cause irritation.

SCALP PSORIASIS

Scalp involvement is very common. Indeed the scalp may be the only

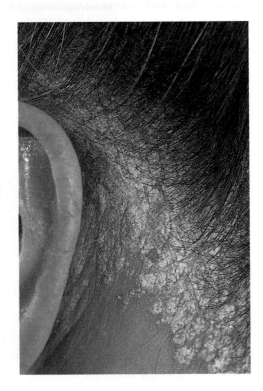

Fig. 8.3 Scalp psoriasis.

affected area. It is sometimes difficult to distinguish scalp psoriasis from severe seborrhoeic dermatitis (see also flexural psoriasis below), but psoriasis is generally thicker. As a rule of thumb, if you can feel scalp lesions as well as see them, they are probably psoriasis.

Lesions vary from one or two plaques to a sheet of thick scale covering the whole scalp surface (Fig. 8.3). Rarely, the scale becomes very thick indeed and sticks in large chunks to bundles of hair. This is known as 'pityriasis amiantacea'. There may be temporary hair loss in severe scalp psoriasis.

NAIL PSORIASIS

Nail abnormalities are frequent, and are one of the most useful diagnostic clues if skin lesions are few, or atypical. Nail changes are almost always present in arthropathic psoriasis.

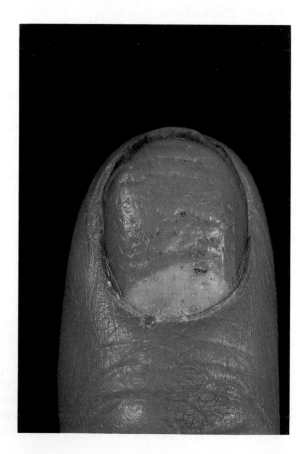

Fig. 8.4 Nail pits in psoriasis.

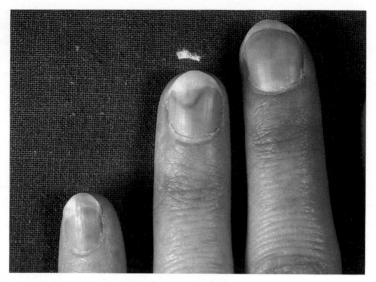

Fig. 8.5 Early psoriatic onycholysis.

There are two common findings which may occur together or alone: pitting and onycholysis. Psoriatic nail pits are relatively large and irregularly arranged (Fig. 8.4), compared with those of alopecia areata. Onycholysis (lifting of the nail plate) initially produces a dull red area with a salmon pink rim (Fig. 8.5). In time, the nail becomes discoloured brown or yellow. It is sometimes painful. These nail changes, particularly onycholysis, may also occur without other evidence of the disease.

Occasionally, pustular changes occur at the ends of the digits and in the nail bed itself (sometimes known as 'acrodermatitis continua'). Similar changes may accompany chronic palmo-plantar pustulosis (see below). In erythrodermic or pustular forms of psoriasis the whole nail surface may become roughened and discoloured.

GUTTATE PSORIASIS

The guttate form of psoriasis often develops suddenly, and may follow an infection, especially a streptococcal sore throat. It is a common way for psoriasis to present, particularly in young adults.

Gutta is the Latin for 'drop'. Most lesions are about a centimetre in diameter (Fig. 8.6), and the colour is usually paler pink than established plaque psoriasis, at least initially. The main differential diagnosis is pityriasis rosea (see Chapter 15), and these disorders are best distinguished by the presence of parakeratotic scale in psoriasis, and the shape of the lesions

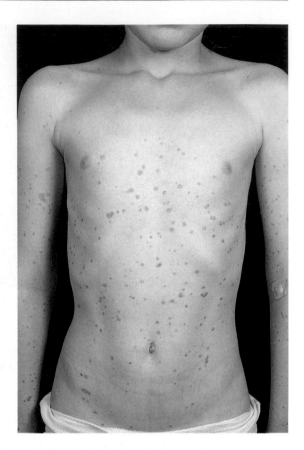

Fig. 8.6 Guttate psoriasis.

(round in guttate psoriasis; oval in pityriasis rosea). Guttate psoriasis may itch.

The lesions of guttate psoriasis often resolve rapidly, but in some patients the patches enlarge and become stable plaques.

FLEXURAL PSORIASIS

Flexural involvement in psoriasis may accompany typical plaque lesions, but is also commonly seen alone, or associated with scalp and nail changes. Lesions may occur in the groin, natal cleft, axillae, umbilicus and sub-mammary folds. Maceration inevitably occurs in these areas, and the surface scale is often lost, leaving a rather beefy erythematous rash (Fig. 8.7). It may be difficult to distinguish this from flexural seborrhoeic dermatitis, so look for nail changes or evidence of psoriasis elsewhere. Some dermatologists consider that there is an overlap state, and call such changes 'sebo-psoriasis'.

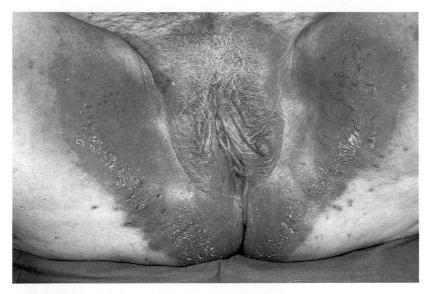

Fig. 8.7 Flexural psoriasis.

Flexural psoriasis is often itchy. Watch out for a secondary contact sensitivity from the use of proprietary anti-itch preparations.

BRITTLE PSORIASIS

Occasionally you will see patients whose psoriasis does not consist of thick, stable plaques, but of thin, irritable scaly areas (Fig. 8.8). Such lesions may arise *de novo* or develop suddenly in a patient whose psoriasis has been stable for years. One reason for this is systemic steroid therapy (often for another condition), and potent topical steroids can also induce stable psoriasis to become 'brittle'.

The significance of brittle psoriasis is that the lesions may rapidly generalize, especially if treated with potent agents (see treatment section below), leading to erythroderma or even acute pustular psoriasis.

ERYTHRODERMIC PSORIASIS

When psoriatic plaques merge to involve most, or all, of the skin a state of erythroderma or exfoliative dermatitis results. The effects of this are discussed in Chapter 15.

Psoriasis may become erythrodermic by slow, inexorable progression, or erythroderma may develop rapidly. Occasionally, erythrodermic psoriasis may appear *de novo*. Systemic steroids or potent topical steroids may precipitate this.

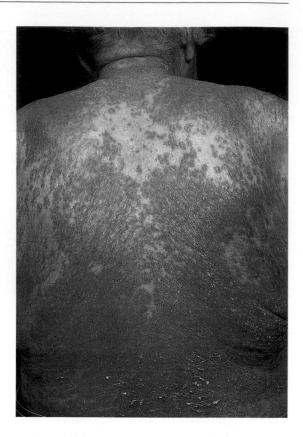

Fig. 8.8 Widespread 'brittle' psoriasis.

ACUTE PUSTULAR PSORIASIS (OF VON ZUMBUSCH)

This is a very serious condition. Patients with or without pre-existing psoriasis suddenly develop widespread erythema. Superimposed on these areas are pustules which may coalesce into lakes of pus (Fig. 8.9). Swabs are sterile.

The patient has a high, swinging fever and is toxic and unwell, with a leucocytosis. If the disease is unchecked, patients become increasingly ill and may die, often of secondary infections.

CHRONIC PALMO-PLANTAR PUSTULOSIS (PUSTULAR PSORIASIS OF PALMS AND SOLES)

There is some debate about the relationship between this condition and other forms of psoriasis. Biopsies reveal psoriasiform pathology, but it is unusual for patients to have chronic palmo-plantar pustulosis in association with other types of psoriatic lesion.

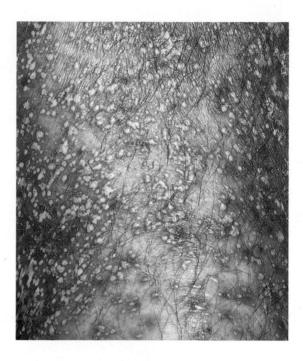

Fig. 8.9 Acute pustular psoriasis.

The typical changes consist of erythematous patches with numerous pustules (Fig. 8.10). These gradually change into brown, scaly spots and peel off. The condition is usually uncomfortable or painful, rather than itchy.

Lesions may involve only a small area of one hand or foot, or cover the entire surface of both palms and soles. This may lead to considerable disability.

THE TREATMENT OF PSORIASIS

The agents most widely used in the treatment of the skin lesions of psoriasis are:

AGENTS FOR TREATING PSORIASIS

Topical
- Emollients
- Tar
- Salicylic acid
- Topical steroids

Continued on p. 110

AGENTS FOR TREATING PSORIASIS
(Continued)

Topical cont.
- Dithranol (anthralin)
- Calcipotriol
- Ultraviolet radiation

Systemic
- PUVA (psoralen + ultraviolet A)
- Retinoids
- Cytotoxics, e.g.:
  methotrexate
  azathioprine
  hydroxyurea
- Systemic steroids
- Cyclosporin

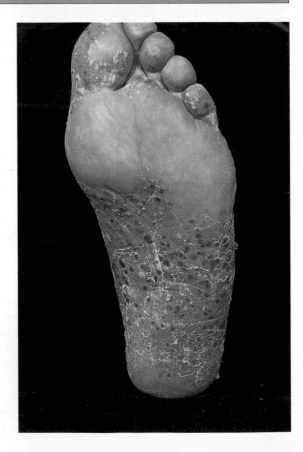

Fig. 8.10 Chronic palmo-plantar pustulosis.

It is an old adage that if there are many treatments for a disease, none works perfectly. This is certainly true of psoriasis. Although each modality is useful in some patients, they all represent a degree of compromise in term of safety, effectiveness or convenience. Many patients require a regimen of different agents for different sites at different times.

TOPICAL THERAPIES

Many agents can be used topically to induce a remission or an improvement. Most are safe, but they are tedious for patients to use, as treatment may have to continue for months or even years.

Emollients

Some patients are prepared to tolerate plaques (especially on covered sites) if the scaling can be controlled. Emollients such as white or yellow soft paraffin or lanolin may accomplish this.

Salicylic acid

Salicylic acid is a 'keratolytic' agent and helps to reduce scaling. It can be used with tar in mixtures, and is also combined with a potent topical steroid in a commercially available preparation.

Tar

Tar has been used for many years, particularly in combination with UV radiation. The most effective preparations are extracts of crude coal tar, often in the form of alcoholic solutions such as liquor picis carbonis. Attempts have been made to refine tar to make it more cosmetically acceptable, but the most effective forms still seem to be the darkest, smelliest and messiest. Consequently, not many patients will use tar for widespread, routine use. However, in bath oils or in ointment mixtures tar may be helpful for skin lesions, and is still valuable in treating scalp disease.

Topical steroids

Topical steroids do not eradicate psoriatic lesions, but may suppress them. Some dermatologists say they never use topical steroids in psoriasis because of the risks (they may induce 'brittle' psoriasis). However, if used with care in stable disease, and on the scalp and in the flexures, they can be useful.

Dithranol (anthralin)

Dithranol can convert psoriatic plaques into completely normal-looking skin. The mode of action is unknown. The 'Ingram regime'—a combination of dithranol, tar and UV radiation—has been used for many years, and patients can be cleared in about 3 weeks of daily treatment. Originally, the dithranol was left on the skin for 24 hours, but this is unnecessary, as 'short-contact' therapy is just as good.

Dithranol seems to work best in Lassar's paste (starch, zinc oxide and salicylic acid in white soft paraffin), but is also available in cream and ointment bases. It is usual to begin with a low concentration (0.1%) and increase this as necessary.

The main complications are staining (due to oxidation to a dye) and burning. Skin staining is temporary, but baths, bedding and clothes may be permanently marked. Dithranol burns can be very unpleasant, especially around the eyes. Patients must be taught to use dithranol carefully.

Calcipotriol

This vitamin D analogue often works very well, and has rapidly found a place in routine management. There are few side-effects, but calcium levels may be disturbed if large quantities are applied.

Ultraviolet Radiation

The use of UV light therapy is well established, the most effective wavelengths being in the medium (UVB) range. UVB must be used with care because it also induces sunburn. Patients require doses which just induce erythema but do not cause burning. The dose is then increased gradually as a tan develops. Treatment is usually given two or three times weekly until clearance is achieved. Adjunctive tar may make the UVB more effective.

UVB is theoretically carcinogenic (as is tar), but surprisingly few psoriasis sufferers develop skin cancers.

SYSTEMIC THERAPIES

Psoralen + ultraviolet A (PUVA)

'Psoralens' form chemical bonds with DNA in the presence of UV radiation. The most widely used agent in the treatment of psoriasis is 8-methoxypsoralen, which is usually taken by mouth 2 hours before exposure to long-wavelength UV light (UVA), initially two to three times weekly. Protective glasses are worn to prevent ocular damage. There is a significant risk of keratoses and epithelial cancers.

Cytotoxic drugs

The most effective and widely used cytotoxic is methotrexate, a folic acid antagonist. Most psoriasis responds to a *once weekly* dose of 7.5–20 mg. Other drugs include azathioprine and hydroxyurea.

All cytotoxics have unwanted effects, particularly bone marrow suppression. This is rare with methotrexate, but may occur in an idiosyncratic manner unrelated to dose. The major problem with methotrexate is hepatotoxicity, particularly fibrosis with chronic use. Alcohol appears to exacerbate this tendency. Younger patients require regular liver biopsies. Methotrexate also inhibits spermatogenesis and is teratogenic. These complications restrict its use to severely affected patients.

Retinoids

Vitamin A derivatives help some patients with psoriasis. The most commonly used is acitretin. Retinoids have a number of cutaneous side-effects, including dry lips, nose-bleeds and hair loss. They may also induce hyperlipidaemia and produce liver function test abnormalities, and they are teratogenic.

Systemic steroids

In very severe psoriasis, steroids may occasionally be necessary, but should not be used alone.

Cyclosporin

This immunosuppressive drug works extremely well, even in very severe psoriasis. It is nephrotoxic and very expensive.

Treatment of clinical patterns of psoriasis

The choice of agent and regimen in psoriasis is dictated by the type and extent of lesions and the effects on the patient's quality of life. A balance will often have to be struck between the need for improvement and the inconvenience and/or side-effects of the agent(s) concerned.

CHRONIC PLAQUE PSORIASIS

Dithranol is a theoretical first choice, but the patient's life-style, or side-effects of the drug, may make it impractical. If so, calcipotriol or topical steroids (with or without tar and salicylic acid) are often used. UV radiation may help. If lesions become very extensive, or if there are serious psychosocial problems, PUVA, retinoids or cytotoxic drugs may be indicated.

SCALP PSORIASIS

Tar shampoos are helpful, but will seldom control thick plaques alone. Tar gels may help, but the best topical remedy is Unguentum Cocois Co.—a mixture including tar and salicylic acid. This is massaged in at night and washed out the following morning. Topical steroid lotions, with or without salicylic acid are also used.

NAIL PSORIASIS

Nail changes do not respond to topical treatment, and systemic drugs are seldom justified for nails alone.

GUTTATE PSORIASIS

This is most easily treated with UV radiation together with a tar-based ointment.

FLEXURAL PSORIASIS

Psoriasis in the flexures poses problems. Mild tar/corticosteroid mixtures may be effective, but long-term use of topical steroids can cause striae. Dithranol, if used in very low concentrations, can be successful, but burning is common and underclothes are stained. UVB and PUVA generally fail to reach the affected areas.

BRITTLE PSORIASIS

Brittle psoriasis requires careful management. Avoid potent topical steroids, strong tar and salicylic acid preparations. Emollients or very dilute steroids may bring the skin into a more stable condition, but PUVA, retinoids or methotrexate may be needed, at least for a short time.

ERYTHRODERMIC AND ACUTE PUSTULAR PSORIASIS

Although both of these states may settle with conservative management, it is more likely that systemic treatment will be required. Such intervention can be life saving. The most common choice is methotrexate, but cyclosporin also works well. When the condition is stable, the dose should be gradually reduced and the drug stopped if possible. However, many patients relapse and require long-term treatment.

CHRONIC PALMO-PLANTAR PUSTULOSIS

Nothing really works well in this condition. Tar pastes, potent topical steroids or dithranol are often ineffective. PUVA to the hands and feet may provide control, but relapse is common.

ARTHROPATHIC PSORIASIS

One of the most unpleasant complications of psoriasis is arthropathy. This may affect up to 10% of psoriatics. There are four basic patterns.

PSORIATIC ARTHROPATHY PATTERNS

- Distal interphalangeal joint involvement
- Seronegative rheumatoid-like joint changes
- Large joint mono-or polyarthropathy
- Spondylitis

The commonest pattern is that involving the distal interphalangeal joints, with the others listed above in descending order of frequency. Psoriatic arthropathy is erosive and may result in joint destruction.

Psoriatics who develop the spondylitic form are usually HLA B27 positive, and there is some overlap between psoriatic arthropathy and other seronegative arthritides.

Treatment involves the judicious use of non-steroidal anti-inflammatory drugs and methotrexate.

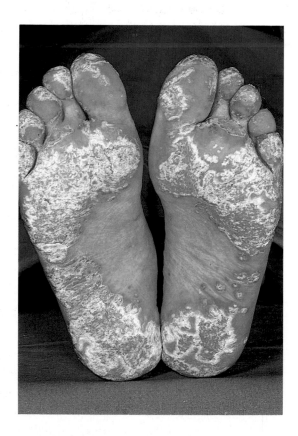

Fig. 8.11 Keratoderma blennorrhagicum.

REITER'S SYNDROME

This disorder, which frequently follows a diarrhoeal illness or non-specific urethritis in HLA B27-positive individuals, is discussed in Chapter 19. Occasionally skin lesions known as 'keratoderma blennorrhagicum' develop. Palmar and plantar lesions may become very gross (Fig. 8.11), and lesions elsewhere are clinically very similar to psoriasis. Histologically, keratoderma blennorrhagicum is indistinguishable from psoriasis.

CHAPTER 9

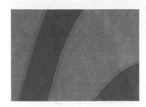

Benign and Malignant Skin Tumours

Know ye not that a little leaven leaveneth the whole lump?
St Paul (1 Corinthians, 5:6)

INTRODUCTION AND CLASSIFICATION OF SKIN TUMOURS

Lumps on or in the skin are extremely common: in our out-patients in Leicester 27% of patients have one of nine common types of skin tumour, and a further 19% have viral warts (see Chapter 3). This workload is rising because:

1 the age of the population as a whole is rising (many skin tumours are commoner in the elderly);

2 skin cancer is increasing in all age groups;

3 there is an increasing public awareness of the importance of skin tumours.

Most skin tumours are benign, often representing only a cosmetic nuisance. However, it is important to distinguish these from malignant or potentially malignant tumours quickly and effectively, as decisions about what can or should be done about a lesion can only be made after a diagnosis to this minimum level has been made.

The skin is a complex organ system, with both benign and malignant tumours described for every component. Table 9.1 presents a simplified version of the wide variety of skin tumours which can occur.

TYPES OF TUMOURS

A Epidermis (for naevi see Chapter 10)

Benign
- Seborrhoeic keratosis
- Skin tags
- Keratoacanthoma
- Clear cell acanthoma (viral warts) (see Chapter 3)
- Tumours of skin appendages, e.g. sweat glands, sebaceous glands, hair follicles
- Epidermal cysts

Dysplastic/malignant
- Basal cell carcinoma
- Actinic (solar) keratosis
- Squamous cell carcinoma:
  in situ (Bowen's disease)
  invasive
- Paget's disease
- Tumours of skin appendages

B Melanocytes (for naevi see Chapter 10)

Benign
- Freckle and lentigo

Dysplastic/malignant
- Dysplastic naevus (see Chapter 10)
- Lentigo maligna
- Malignant melanoma:
  lentigo maligna melanoma
  superficial spreading
  nodular
  acral

C Dermis (for naevi see Chapter 10)

Benign
- Fibrous tissue:
  dermatofibroma
- 'Neural' tissue e.g.:
  e.g. neurofibroma

Table 9.1 Tumours, benign or malignant, found in the epidermis and dermis.

TYPES OF TUMOURS

- Vascular tissue:
  angioma/angiokeratoma
  pyogenic granuloma
  glomus tumour

Dysplastic/malignant
- Fibrosarcoma
- Neurofibrosarcoma
- Angiosarcoma, including Kaposi's sarcoma

D Pseudo-tumours
- Chondrodermatitis nodularis helicis
- Hypertrophic and keloid scars

E Lymphomata
- Cutaneous T cell lymphoma (mycosis fungoides)
- Cutaneous B cell lymphoma

F Extension from deeper tissues

G Metastatic deposits

Table 9.1 *Continued.*

GENERAL TREATMENT PRINCIPLES FOR SKIN TUMOURS

It is worth reviewing briefly the techniques which may be used to treat skin tumours. This will avoid repetition.

The first important principle is that, unless the diagnosis is certain, some tissue should be preserved for histology. Failure to do this will mean missed malignancies, and is one explanation for patients who present with mysterious lymphatic or distant deposits from unknown primary sites.

Surgical removal or biopsy

These techniques have already been described and illustrated (Figs 2.1 and 2.2). Removal of small skin tumours is quick, simple and economical. If the tumour is too large for primary excision, take a small incisional biopsy, remembering to cross the edge from normal to abnormal tissue. There is no evidence that such a biopsy adversely affects the outcome, although incisional biopsy of invasive melanomas should be avoided if possible (see below).

Curettage and/or cautery ('C&C')

This is a perfectly satisfactory method for removal of superficial tumours.

C & C

1 Use a curette (Volkmann spoon) to scrape lesions off
2 Touch the raw base a few times with the cautery to control oozing
3 Apply a simple dressing and/or antiseptic

An alternative to cautery is a hyfrecator—a machine which produces electrical haemostasis and desiccation.

Pedunculated tumours can be removed by slicing with cautery across the base.

Cryotherapy

The use of cryotherapy for tumours has become very popular. It is ideal for superficial skin tumours because it is quick and leaves relatively little scarring. However, histological interpretation of cryobiopsies is not easy and it should be used only if: the tumour is definitely benign; or an incisional biopsy has already been performed. Cryotherapy is not appropriate for melanomas.

The best agent for cryotherapy is liquid nitrogen.

CRYOTHERAPY

1 Apply nitrogen with cotton-wool buds, or by specially designed spray or probe instruments
2 Wait until a halo of frozen skin 1 mm around the tumour is obtained
3 Maintain halo for 10 seconds for benign, 30 seconds for malignant tumours
4 Allow to thaw, and repeat (two 'freeze/thaw cycles')

The patient should be told to expect blistering, followed by healing with crust formation. The lesion should separate within 3 weeks.

Radiotherapy

Radiotherapy is an effective method for the treatment of basal and squamous cell carcinomas, and is often the most practical option for very large tumours in the elderly. However, it is not ideal for some areas of the body, and the choice between excision and radiotherapy should be based on individual circumstances.

Radiotherapy can also control secondary tumour deposits to some extent.

SPECIFIC TUMOURS

We shall first consider benign tumours, and then dysplastic and malignant processes, discussing the commonest and most important of these.

Some skin lumps are hamartomatous malformations. Such a lesion in the skin is termed a 'naevus'. Naevi are discussed separately in Chapter 10.

Benign tumours—epidermal

SEBORRHOEIC KERATOSES (SEBORRHOEIC WARTS; BASAL CELL PAPILLOMAS)

You are bound to see some seborrhoeic keratoses, if only in passing while examining a chest. They are most frequent in the elderly, and may be solitary or multiple. Occasionally there are hundreds of lesions, a tendency which may be familial.

Clinical features: a flat-topped area of skin with a 'stuck-on' appearance (Fig. 9.1). They may be pale, but are often pigmented, sometimes deeply so. The surface is often said to be 'greasy', but a more useful sign is small surface pits and irregularities, giving the surface a granular look.

Sites of predilection: head and neck; backs of hands and forearms; trunk.

Differential diagnosis: usually straightforward, but darkly pigmented lesions can be mistaken for melanomas. On the face, seborrhoeic keratoses may remain virtually flat, causing difficulty in distinguishing them from senile lentigo or lentigo maligna (see below). Another diagnostic problem arises if lesions become inflamed as a result of external trauma. There may be crusting and bleeding, and biopsy for histology may be necessary.

Treatment: if deemed necessary (there is no malignant potential), the best approach for smaller lesions is cryotherapy. Larger ones may be better treated by curettage and cautery or excision.

SKIN TAGS (ACROCHORDONS)

Many people develop these small pedunculated lesions around the neck and in the axillae. Increasing age and obesity are predisposing factors.

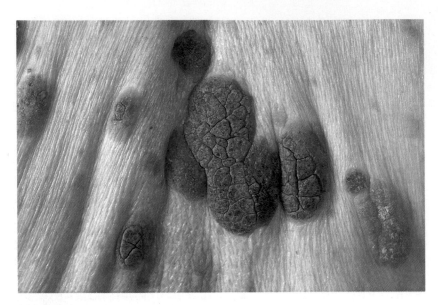

Fig. 9.1 Typical seborrhoeic warts.

Differential diagnosis: small melanocytic naevi may look similar, and so may small pedunculated seborrhoeic keratoses.

Treatment: they can be removed very easily with a cautery.

KERATOACANTHOMA (ONCE CALLED 'MOLLUSCUM SEBACEUM')

This tumour is an oddity. Some authors classify keratoacanthoma as malignant because the histology resembles a squamous cell carcinoma (see below). Keratoacanthomas are much commoner in the elderly.

Clinical features: lesions arise rapidly, reaching a maximal size over the course of 6–8 weeks (Fig. 9.2). The tumour is round, with rolled edges and a central keratin plug. The base is often red and inflamed, and may be painful. Ultimately, the tumour begins to shrink, often almost as quickly as it enlarged, and disappears completely, leaving a small puckered scar.

Sites of predilection: almost invariably on light-exposed skin.

Differential diagnosis: differentiation from basal cell carcinoma (see below) can be made on the basis of the history of rapid growth and on the perfect roundness of the lesion.

The main problem is to distinguish *prospectively* between a keratoacanthoma and a squamous cell carcinoma. By definition a keratoacanthoma should resolve spontaneously, but this cannot be determined in advance.

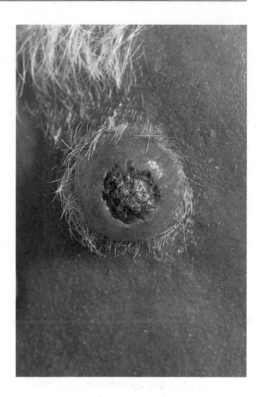

Fig. 9.2 Keratoacanthoma.

Incisional biopsies do not help because of the close similarities to squamous cell carcinoma.

   Treatment: it is reasonable to wait expectantly for a short while if a lesion is very typical, especially in the elderly or frail. However, if there is any diagnostic doubt keratoacanthomas are best removed and sent for histology. There is a case for removing such a lesion early, in order to avoid the necessity for a more complex procedure if it becomes much larger.

OTHER BENIGN EPIDERMAL TUMOURS

Viral warts are discussed in Chapter 3, and the other benign epidermal tumours listed are rare.

EPIDERMAL CYSTS

There are three common forms of epidermal cyst—pilar, epidermoid, and milium.

   I Common scalp cysts are correctly termed 'pilar' or 'trichilemmal' cysts.

There may be several, and a familial predisposition to develop these cysts is usual.

2 Epidermoid cysts may be found anywhere, but are most common on the head, neck and trunk. They often follow severe acne; there is a cystic swelling within the skin, usually with an overlying punctum.

   Treatment: both types can be removed easily under local anaesthetic using a linear incision over the surface.

3 Milia are extremely common keratin cysts, which may occur spontaneously or after trauma or blistering. In some families there is an inherited tendency to develop clusters on the cheeks and around the eyes (Fig. 9.3).

   Treatment: milia can be treated by incision, pricking out or cautery.

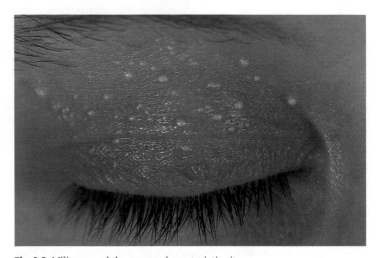

Fig. 9.3 Milia around the eyes: a characteristic site.

Benign melanocytic tumours

FRECKLES (EPHELIDES) AND LENTIGINES

Freckles are areas of skin containing melanocytes which are normal in number but are hyper-responsive to ultraviolet radiation. They are genetically determined: we are all familiar with freckly red-headed individuals.

   Lentigines are flat pigmented areas composed of increased numbers of melanocytes.

   Melanocytic naevi are discussed in Chapter 10.

Benign tumours—dermal

DERMATOFIBROMA (OR HISTIOCYTOMA)

Dermatofibromas (Fig. 9.4) are composed of fibrous tissue and some blood vessels. It is not known why they occur, but they may follow minor trauma.

Clinical features: more common in women; often easier to diagnose by touch than by sight: they feel like small lentils.

Sites of predilection: usually found on the legs.

Differential diagnosis: occasionally, heavy pigmentation can cause confusion with melanoma.

Treatment: excision may be cosmetically indicated.

ANGIOMA

Angiomas of various kinds are seen. They are collections of aberrant blood vessels within the dermis and/or subcutaneous tissues. Some are develop-

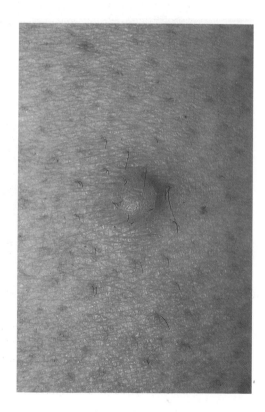

Fig. 9.4 Dermatofibroma (histiocytoma).

mental defects, commonly present at birth, and these are discussed in Chapter 10. Others develop during adult life, such as the ubiquitous Campbell de Morgan spots (Fig. 9.5).

PYOGENIC GRANULOMA

Pyogenic granulomata are benign reactive inflammatory masses composed of blood vessels with a few fibroblasts.

Clinical features: they erupt rapidly and usually have a polypoid appearance (Fig. 9.6), and a 'collar' around the base; profuse contact bleeding is a common presenting symptom.

Sites of predilection: sites of an injury or infection, often on a digit.

Differential diagnosis: they must be differentiated from squamous cell carcinomas and amelanotic melanomas.

Treatment: removal by curettage or excision should **always** be followed by histological examination.

OTHERS

You may encounter several other benign dermal or subcutaneous lumps: neurofibromas, e.g. in von Recklinghausen's neurofibromatosis (see Chapter 11); various benign fibroblastic tumours; lipomata, which are readily identified by their soft texture and lobulated outline.

If there is any doubt about any dermal or subcutaneous lump it is best removed for histology.

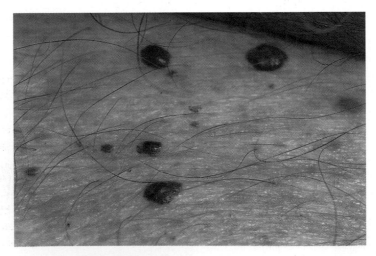

Fig. 9.5 Campbell de Morgan spots.

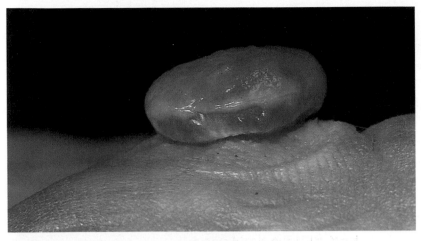

Fig. 9.6 Side-view of a typical pyogenic granuloma.

PSEUDO-TUMOURS

Chondrodermatitis nodularis helicis

This curious lesion is not a tumour, but an inflammatory process.

Clinical features: a small umbilicated nodule on the rim of the ear, usually in men (Fig. 9.7); the clue is that it is painful, especially in bed at night.

Differential diagnosis: it is often confused with basal cell carcinomas or other tumours.

Treatment: it can easily be excised.

Hypertrophic scars and keloids

Scar formation can become very exuberant, especially in some sites (see below) and in children, young adults and black skin. Some authors only use the term 'keloid' for lesions which spread laterally beyond the original site (keloids can become very large).

Clinical features: protuberant masses of fibrous tissue usually following trauma: cuts (which may be surgical), ear-piercing, burns, acne, Bacille Calmette–Guérin (BCG) inoculations (if performed high on the shoulder); some appear to develop spontaneously; keloids often itch.

Sites of predilection: chest, upper back, shoulder, pubic region, ear lobes.

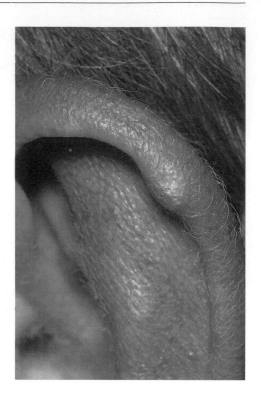

Fig. 9.7 Chondrodermatitis nodularis helicis.

Differential diagnosis: any soft tissue tumour, especially if there is no preceding history of trauma.

Treatment: excision generally leads to recurrence, and management can be extremely difficult. Intralesional steroids, cryotherapy, and radiotherapy before and after excision all have their advocates.

DYSPLASTIC AND MALIGNANT TUMOURS

The term 'dysplasia' implies that the skin has been partly or wholly replaced by cells which show neoplastic features. When this results in invasion of adjacent tissue, the process can genuinely be said to be 'malignant'.

Cutaneous dysplasias and malignancies are increasingly common, especially in ageing skin and in skin exposed to prolonged UV radiation. Other factors are also associated with dysplastic skin changes:

1 most forms of ionizing radiation (UV light, X-rays, γ-rays) are powerful inducers of skin cancer;

2 there are a number of known carcinogens: exposure to some industrial oils, tars and bitumen; exposure to soot in chimney sweeps used to result in scrotal cancers;

3 skin cancers are a feature of some genetic diseases: a notable example is xeroderma pigmentosum, in which the repair of UV-induced DNA damage is faulty.

Dysplastic/malignant epidermal tumours

BASAL CELL CARCINOMA (BCC)

The commonest malignant skin tumour is often known as a 'rodent ulcer'.

Clinical features: most begin as a nodule (Fig. 9.8) which spreads slowly outwards, usually leaving a central depression (this creates the classical 'rolled edge'); tumours are usually skin-coloured with a translucent look (often described as 'pearly'); telangiectatic vessels on the surface are very characteristic, and account for the frequent presenting complaint of contact bleeding; metastasis is extremely rare, but local invasion can be very destructive (Fig. 9.9) and BCCs can spread along bony passages into the skull.

Variants: several distinctive clinical variants of the BCC are recognized (see p. 130):

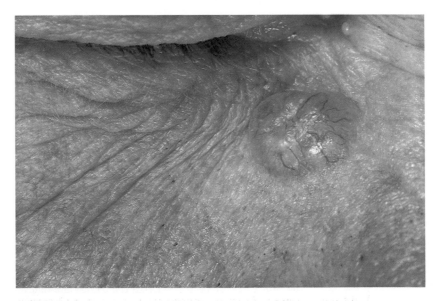

Fig. 9.8 Basal cell carcinoma. Note the telangiectatic vessels.

CLINICAL VARIANTS

Morphoeic
A flat growth pattern which results in a scar-like appearance; it can be very difficult to know where the tumour begins and ends, and local invasion is more common

Superficial
Lesions grow for many years and may be many centimetres across; usually solitary; multiple tumours may indicate previous arsenic ingestion; characteristically, a 'worm-like' edge is seen (Fig. 9.10)

Pigmented
Pigmentation is usually patchy but may be very dark and dense

Sites of predilection: predominantly the face, but BCCs occur on other sun-exposed sites, in the hair-bearing scalp, behind the ear, and on the trunk (where the superficial pattern is common).

Differential diagnosis: early lesions may be confused with naevi; superficial BCCs are often treated as inflammatory; heavy pigmentation may suggest a melanoma; morphoeic tumours can be very difficult to diagnose.

Treatment: excision, biopsy and radiotherapy or, for superficial tumours, curettage or cryotherapy; careful assessment of morphoeic tumours is needed—a technique known as 'microscopically controlled surgery' may be helpful; it is particularly important to deal adequately with lesions around the eyes, nose and ears.

ACTINIC OR SOLAR KERATOSES

These are areas of dysplastic squamous epithelium without invasion, but actinic keratoses do have low-grade malignant potential and their presence indicates unstable epithelium.

Clinical features: red and scaly patches (Fig. 9.11) which characteristically wax and wane with time; many hundreds of lesions may occur in heavily sun-exposed individuals.

Sites of predilection: light-exposed skin, especially the face, forearms, dorsa of hands, lower legs and bald scalp.

Differential diagnosis: some are pigmented, leading to confusion with lentigo maligna (see below).

Treatment: cryotherapy is best for small numbers of lesions; large areas on the face and scalp can be treated with the topical anti-mitotic agent 5-fluorouracil; in the very elderly it may be best to do nothing.

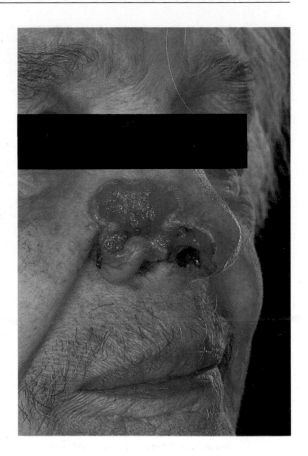

Fig. 9.9 Basal cell carcinoma. Such destruction gives rise to the term 'rodent ulcer'.

SQUAMOUS CELL CARCINOMA (SCC) *IN SITU* (OR BOWEN'S DISEASE)

Bowen's disease is a SCC confined to the epidermis, and is common in the elderly. Invasive change does occur but is rare.

Clinical features: usually solitary patch of red scaly skin, although multiple areas may occur; Bowen's disease is asymptomatic.

Variant: erythroplasia of Queyrat—non-invasive dysplastic changes may also occur on the penis, where the clinical appearance is of a velvety red plaque. Although given a separate name, it is essentially the same as Bowen's disease elsewhere.

Sites of predilection: light-exposed skin; may occur on non-exposed areas such as the trunk.

Differential diagnosis: there is a superficial resemblance to psoriasis

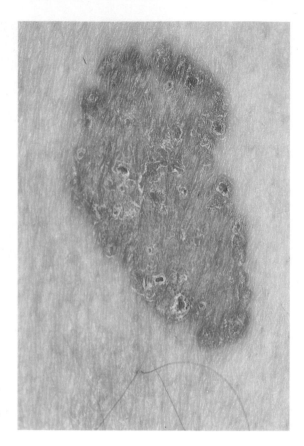

Fig. 9.10 Superficial basal cell carcinoma.

(Fig. 9.12), but the surface scale is adherent rather than flaky. Removal of scale leaves a glistening red surface which does not bleed. As arsenic was used in the past to treat psoriasis, keep an eye out for Bowen's disease in elderly psoriasis sufferers.

Similar changes on one nipple should always suggest the possibility of *Paget's disease* (Fig. 9.13); a biopsy should be performed as there is always an underlying carcinoma.

Treatment: should be treated by curettage or cryotherapy; very large areas may require radiotherapy.

INVASIVE SQUAMOUS CELL CARCINOMA

SCCs are locally invasive, and may metastasize to regional lymph nodes

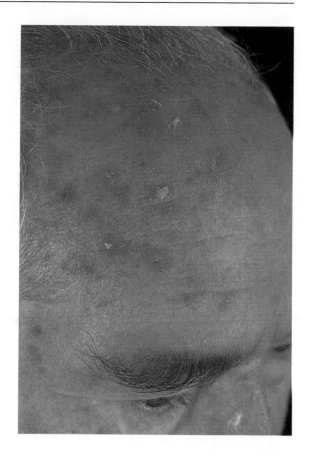

Fig. 9.11 Multiple solar keratoses.

and beyond (especially lip, mouth and genital lesions). UV radiation is important aetiologically, but other factors also play a role: smoking in lip and mouth cancers; wart virus in genital lesions.

Clinical features: may be very varied, typically either:

1 a keratotic lump;

2 a rapidly growing polypoid mass (Fig. 9.14);

3 a cutaneous ulcer.

SCCs are often surrounded by actinic keratoses.

Sites of predilection: sun-exposed sites; SCCs also develop on the lips, in the mouth (Fig. 9.15) and on the genitalia.

Differential diagnosis: keratotic lesions may closely resemble hypertrophic actinic keratoses.

Treatment: biopsy of any suspicious lesion; definitive treatment is by surgical removal or radiotherapy.

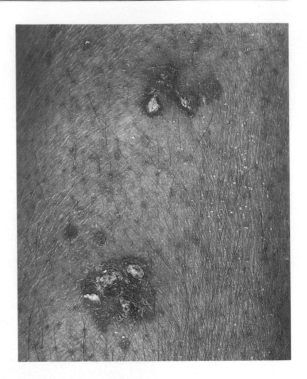

Fig. 9.12 Two patches of Bowen's disease.

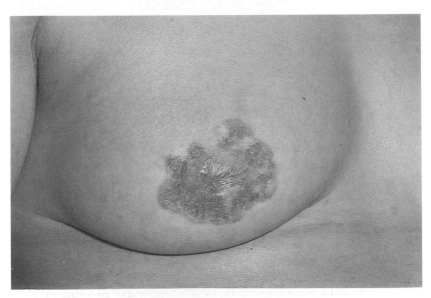

Fig. 9.13 Paget's disease of the nipple.

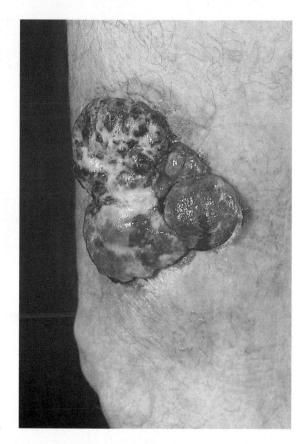

Fig. 9.14 A polypoid squamous cell carcinoma.

Dysplastic/malignant melanocytic tumours

LENTIGO MALIGNA (OR HUTCHINSON'S MALIGNANT FRECKLE)

The term 'lentigo maligna' describes a patch of malignant melanocytes, in sun-damaged skin, which proliferate radially along the dermoepidermal junction, often for many years. An invasive component may develop at any time.

Clinical features: a flat, brown area with irregular pigmentation.

Sites of predilection: almost always on the face (Fig. 9.16).

Differential diagnosis: can be difficult to distinguish from flat seborrhoeic keratoses, pigmented actinic keratoses and simple lentigines.

Treatment: biopsy is essential; definitive treatment is a matter of

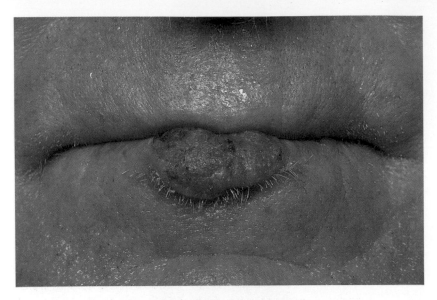

Fig. 9.15 Squamous cell carcinoma on the lip.

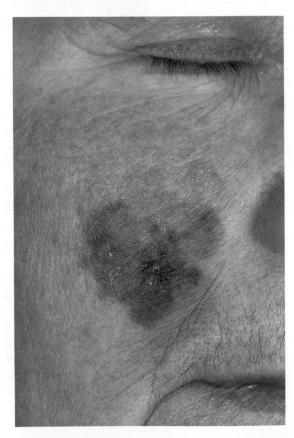

Fig. 9.16 Lentigo maligna.

debate; excision is our preferred option because of recurrences with cryotherapy; in the very elderly it may be reasonable to do nothing and follow the patient carefully.

MALIGNANT MELANOMA (MM)

This is the most dangerous of the malignant skin tumours. Melanomas, other than lentigo maligna melanoma (see below), occur in a relatively younger age group than other skin cancers. The incidence is rising rapidly, even in temperate climates, probably due to the increase in intermittent sun exposure which is now so fashionable. Rising standards of living have permitted more sunny holidays abroad (and at home), during which the most important 'activity' is sunbathing.

Such periods of exposure to strong sunlight (and sunburn) are particularly risky. There is also evidence that childhood sun exposure may be important. It is also important to note that some melanomas arise in pre-existing melanocytic naevi (see Chapter 10). It seems that the incidence of this varies from country to country.

There are four recognized patterns of malignant melanoma.

Treatment of malignant melanoma

In understanding MM and its treatment it is important to realize that the

---

MALIGNANT MELANOMA PATTERNS

Lentigo maligna melanoma
The appearance of a nodule of invasive melanoma within a lentigo maligna.

Superficial spreading melanoma (SSM)
The commonest in the UK; the tumour has a radial growth phase before true invasion begins
- Clinical features:
  irregularly pigmented brown/black patch with an irregular edge (Fig. 9.17)
  may itch or give rise to mild discomfort
  may bleed
- Sites of predilection:
  most frequently on the leg in women and the trunk in men, but may occur anywhere
- Differential diagnosis:
  naevi in the young
  flat seborrhoeic keratoses in older patients

Continued on p. 138

MALIGNANT MELANOMA PATTERNS (Continued)

Nodular melanoma
The tumour exhibits an invasive growth pattern from the outset
- Clinical features:
  rapidly growing lumps (Fig. 9.18)
  occasionally warty (verrucous melanoma) or non-pigmented
  (amelanotic melanoma)
- Sites of predilection:
  may occur anywhere
- Differential diagnosis:
  other rapidly growing tumours

Acral melanoma
Rare in the UK, but is much more common in other countries (e.g. Japan); it is virtually the only type of melanoma seen in Asian or Afro-Caribbean patients
- Clinical features:
  a pigmented patch on the sole or palm or
  an area of subungual pigmentation
- Differential diagnosis:
  can be confused with a viral wart
  must be distinguished from haematoma

Some MMs arise in pre-existing melanocytic naevi, although estimates of the frequency of this vary from 5–10% to over 50%.

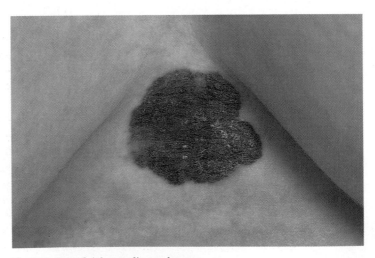

Fig. 9.17 Superficial spreading melanoma.

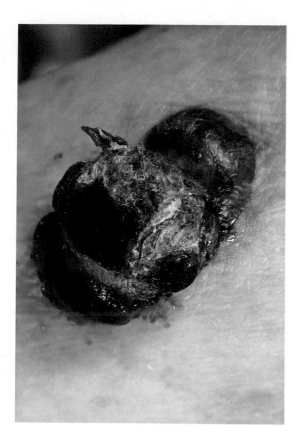

Fig. 9.18 Large nodular melanoma.

prognosis is related to the depth of tumour invasion at first excision, regardless of the original type. Most centres measure invasion using a technique known as the 'Breslow thickness' (Fig. 9.19). If the tumour is less than 1.5 mm at first excision 5-year survival is about 90%; if the depth is over 3.5 mm this falls to 40% or less.

The treatment of all types of melanoma is therefore excision at the earliest possible opportunity. Radiotherapy and chemotherapy have little to offer at present. There is some debate about how wide the excision margins should be, and practice varies from surgeon to surgeon. In general, however, margins are becoming narrower. There is certainly no harm in initial narrow excision. The urgency is to remove the melanoma and consider further procedures later.

In acral melanoma it may be necessary to perform a confirmatory biopsy before definitive treatment, which may involve amputation.

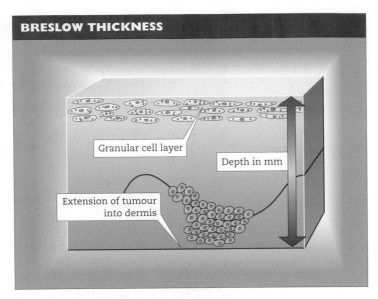

BRESLOW THICKNESS

Granular cell layer

Depth in mm

Extension of tumour
into dermis

Fig. 9.19 Breslow thickness.

Encouraging early presentation

The most effective way of improving treatment is to increase public awareness of MMs and thereby prompt people to seek advice about suspicious
lesions. Many doctors now use a checklist.

MALIGNANT MELANOMA CHECKLIST

- Is an existing mole getting larger or a new one growing? After puberty
  moles usually do not grow. (This sign essentially refers to adults.
  Remember that naevi may grow rapidly in children (see Chapter 10))
- Does the lesion have an irregular outline? Ordinary moles are a smooth,
  regular shape
- Is the lesion irregularly pigmented? Particularly, is there a mixture of
  shades of brown and black?
- Is the lesion larger than 1 cm in diameter?
- Is the lesion inflamed or is there a reddish edge?
- Is the lesion bleeding, oozing or crusting?
- Does the lesion itch or hurt?

Any pigmented lesion, whether newly arising or already present, which
exhibits three or more of the seven listed features, and especially one of
the first three, should be treated as highly suspicious

Prevention of epithelial and melanocytic malignancies

Both types of epithelial skin cancers, and melanomas, are more common in those who burn easily in the sun: those with fair skin, fair or red hair and blue or green eyes (skin types I and II—see Chapter 12). Melanomas are also more common in individuals with many melanocytic naevi.

However, chronic exposure to UV radiation is associated with BCCs and SCCs, and (as mentioned above) most evidence now also links melanoma to UV radiation. It is logical, therefore, to recommend that those at risk avoid excessive sun exposure:

1 no-one should allow themselves to be sunburnt;

2 it is best to avoid midday sun (between 11 a.m. and 3 p.m.) or, at least, wear adequate clothing and hats;

3 sun-screens offering a high degree of protection should be used.

Those who tan easily and those with brown or black skin need not

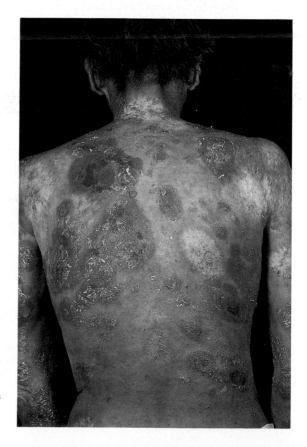

Fig. 9.20 Areas of mycosis fungoides (cutaneous T cell lymphoma).

take such Draconian precautions, but sun exposure in all children should be restricted.

Dermal malignant tumours

Malignant sarcomas may develop in the skin.

Clinical features: indolent, slow-growing nodules, which become fixed to deeper tissues.

Differential diagnosis: difficult to categorize without biopsy.

Treatment: wide excision is generally required; in one tumour of this kind—dermatofibrosarcoma protuberans—very wide indeed.

KAPOSI'S SARCOMA

This malignant vascular tumour merits special mention in spite of its rarity. 'Classical' Kaposi's sarcoma occurs in Ashkenazi Jews and northern Italians. A much more aggressive form is seen in Africans and in patients with the acquired immunodeficiency syndrome (AIDS).

Clinical features: purplish plaques and nodules.

Sites of predilection: legs in the classical form; anywhere in the aggressive form.

Differential diagnosis: other vascular lesions.

Treatment: biopsy; symptomatic treatment with radiotherapy.

LYMPHOMAS

Lymphomatous involvement of the skin may be secondary, e.g. in non-Hodgkin's B cell lymphoma. However, the skin may be the original site, especially in cutaneous T cell lymphoma (often called 'mycosis fungoides').

Clinical features: variable; some areas remain unchanged or grow slowly for years; red, well-circumscribed, scaly plaques and tumours eventually develop (Fig. 9.20).

Differential diagnosis: lesions can be confused with eczema or psoriasis.

Treatment: biopsy is essential; definitive treatment varies with the stage, but includes radiotherapy, PUVA and chemotherapy.

Extension from deeper tissues and metastases

Tumours of underlying structures, such as breast, may invade the skin. The skin may also be the site of metastatic deposits from internal cancers such as bronchogenic carcinoma (see Chapter 19).

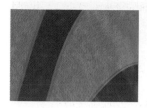

Naevi

Ten thousand saw I at a glance
Wordsworth

INTRODUCTION

Naevi are extremely common—virtually everyone has some. However, the word 'naevus' can give rise to confusion. Much of the difficulty is due to the term being used in several different ways, in addition to that outlined below. Some writers use the word without qualification for the commonest cutaneous haemartoma, the melanocytic naevus (see below). The word is also applied to lesions which are not congenital at all, such as the 'spider naevus' (which should be a 'spider telangiectasis'). This is complicated further by some true 'naevi' being called 'moles' or 'birthmarks': a lump described as a 'mole' may be a melanocytic naevus, but may also be any small skin lesion, especially if pigmented; 'birthmark' is accurate enough as far as it goes, but many true naevi develop after birth.

We use the word 'naevus' to mean a cutaneous haemartoma (a lesion in which normal tissue components are present in abnormal quantities or patterns). This encompasses 'naevi' which are not actually present at birth, because the cells from which they arise are.

Any component of the skin may produce a naevus, and they may be classified accordingly (Table 10.1).

NAEVI CLASSIFICATION

Epithelial/'organoid'
- Epidermal naevus
- Sebaceous naevus
- Hair follicle naevus

Melanocytic

Congenital
- Congenital melanocytic naevus
- Mongolian blue spot

Acquired
- Junctional/compound/intradermal naevus
- Sutton's halo naevus
- Dysplastic naevus
- Spitz naevus
- Blue naevus

Vascular

Telangiectatic
- Superficial capillary naevus
- Deep capillary naevus
- Rare telangiectatic disorders

Angiomatous

Other tissues
- Connective tissue
- Mast cell
- Fat

Table 10.1 A classification of naevi.

We need only discuss the most important: epithelial and organoid naevi, vascular naevi and melanocytic naevi.

EPITHELIAL AND 'ORGANOID' NAEVI

These are relatively uncommon developmental defects of epidermal structures: the epidermis itself; hair follicles; sebaceous glands. There are two important types, the epidermal naevus and the sebaceous naevus.

Epidermal naevus

Circumscribed areas of epidermal thickening may be present at birth or

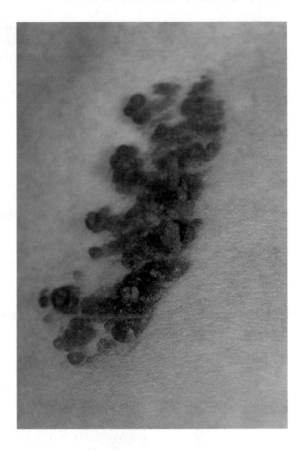

Fig. 10.1 Linear warty
epidermal naevus.

develop during childhood. Many are linear (Fig. 10.1).Very rarely, there are
associated central nervous system (CNS) abnormalities.

Another epidermal naevus is *Becker's naevus*, which is a pigmented
hairy patch first seen at or around puberty on the upper trunk or
shoulder.

Sebaceous naevus

Sebaceous naevi are easily overlooked at birth. Flat, slightly yellow areas
on the head and neck are seen which, in hairy scalp, may cause
localized alopecia. Later, the naevus becomes thickened and warty,
and basal cell carcinomas may arise. They are best excised during
adolescence.

MELANOCYTIC NAEVI

The commonest naevi are formed from melanocytes which have failed to mature or migrate properly during embryonic development. Almost all of us have some. Look at your own skin to see typical examples!

It is convenient to categorize melanocytic naevi by clinical and histopathological features, because there are relevant differences (see Table 10.1). The first is whether they are present at birth (congenital) or arise later (acquired).

Congenital

CONGENITAL MELANOCYTIC NAEVUS

About 1% of children have a melanocytic naevus at birth.

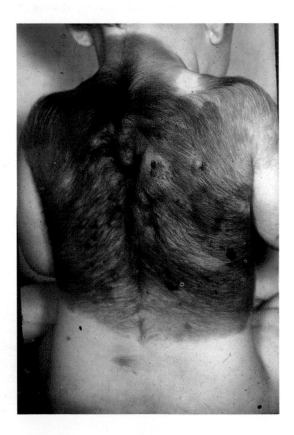

Fig. 10.2 Giant congenital melanocytic naevus.

These vary from a few millimetres to many centimetres in diameter. There is a rare, but huge and grossly disfiguring variant, the 'giant' congenital melanocytic or 'bathing trunk' naevus (Fig. 10.2).

Congenital melanocytic naevi are more prone to develop melanomas than acquired lesions, and this is particularly true of the giant type. Pre-pubertal malignant melanoma is extremely rare, but nearly always involves a congenital naevus. This leads to a paradox: small, low-risk naevi are easily removed but larger lesions with higher malignant potential require extensive, even mutilating, surgery. Each case must be judged on its own merits, and decisions must involve the family.

MONGOLIAN BLUE SPOT

Almost all children of Mongoloid extraction and many Indian and black babies are born with a diffuse blue–black patch on the lower back and buttocks (Fig. 10.3). There are melanocytes widely dispersed in the dermis (the depth is responsible for the colour). The area fades as the child grows up, but may persist indefinitely. Unwary doctors have mistaken Mongolian blue spots for bruising, and accused parents of baby-battering.

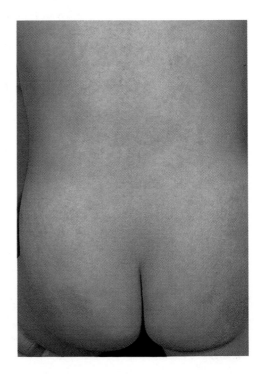

Fig. 10.3 Mongolian blue spot.

ACQUIRED MELANOCYTIC NAEVUS

A melanocytic naevus is 'acquired' if it develops during post-natal life, a phenomenon which is so common as to be 'normal'. Most only represent a minor nuisance, and 'beauty spots' were once highly fashionable.

The first thing to understand is that each naevus has its own life history. This will make the terms applied to the different stages in their evolution clearer (Fig. 10.4).

The lesion (Fig. 10.5) is first noticed when immature melanocytes begin to proliferate at the dermoepidermal junction (hence 'junctional'). After a variable period of radial growth, some cells migrate vertically into the dermis ('compound'). Eventually all melanocytic cells are within the dermis ('intradermal'). Different melanocytic naevi will be at different stages of development in the same individual.

The majority of melanocytic naevi appear in the first 20 years of life, but may continue to develop well into the 40s. They are initially pigmented, often heavily, but later may become pale, especially when intradermal. Most disappear altogether: very few octogenarians have many.

Their importance (apart from cosmetic) is threefold: some malignant melanomas develop in a pre-existing naevus (the chances of this occurring in any one lesion are infinitesimally small); the possession of large numbers

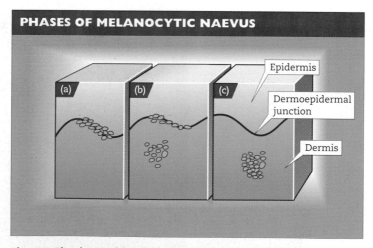

PHASES OF MELANOCYTIC NAEVUS

Epidermis

Dermoepidermal junction

Dermis

Fig. 10.4 The phases of the acquired melanocytic naevus: (a) junctional; (b) compound; and (c) intradermal. These stages are part of a continuum, and each lasts a variable time.

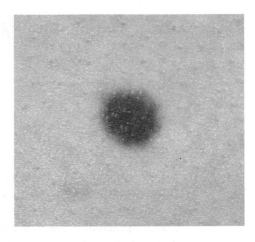

Fig. 10.5 Acquired melanocytic naevus.

of acquired melanocytic naevi is a risk factor for melanoma; and melanocytic naevi can be confused with melanomas clinically.

Any melanocytic lesion which behaves oddly should be excised and examined histologically, but remember that, by definition, all melanocytic naevi grow at some stage. Growth alone, therefore, is not necessarily sinister, especially in younger individuals. Most naevi undergoing malignant change show features outlined in Chapter 9 (p. 140). But . . . if in doubt 'lop it out'!

There are several variants of the acquired melanocytic naevus.

ACQUIRED MELANOCYTIC NAEVUS

Sutton's halo naevus
A white ring develops around an otherwise typical melanocytic naevus; the lesion may become red and disappear (Fig. 10.6). This is an immune response of no sinister significance and unknown cause

Dysplastic naevus
Some lesions look unusual and/or have unusual histopathological features; this may affect just one or two naevi, but some people have many; such individuals may be part of a pedigree in which there is a striking increase in melanoma ('dysplastic naevus syndrome')

Blue naevus
The characteristic slate-blue colour (Fig. 10.7) is due to deep dermal melanocytes; they are most common on the extremities, head and buttocks

Continued on p. 150

ACQUIRED MELANOCYTIC NAEVUS
(Continued)

Spitz naevus
Sometimes called juvenile melanoma with or without the prefix 'benign';
benign lesions, in children have a characteristic brick-red colour; Spitz
naevi can be confused histologically with malignant melanoma

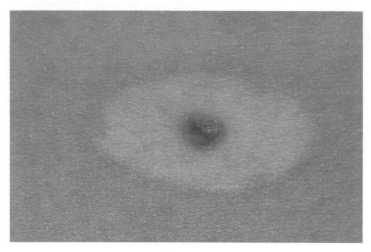

Fig. 10.6 Sutton's 'halo' naevus.

VASCULAR NAEVI

Vascular blemishes are common. Some present relatively minor problems,
whereas others are very disfiguring. The classification of these naevi is confusing and by no means uniform. We have adopted a simple approach based
on both clinical and pathological features.

Telangiectatic naevi

SUPERFICIAL CAPILLARY NAEVUS

These pink, flat areas, composed of dilated capillaries in the superficial
dermis (Fig. 10.8), are found in 50% of neonates. The commonest sites are
the nape of the neck ('salmon patches' or 'stork marks'), the forehead and
glabellar region ('stork marks' again) and the eyelids ('angel's kisses'). Most
facial lesions fade, but those on the neck persist, often hidden by hair.

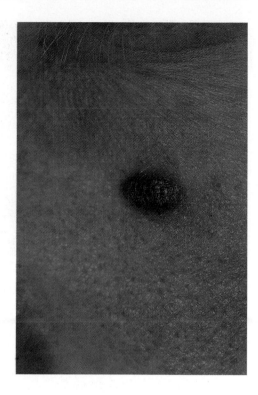

Fig. 10.7 Blue naevus.

DEEP CAPILLARY NAEVUS

'Port-wine stains' or 'port-wine marks' are formed by capillaries in the upper and deeper dermis. The deeper component gradually extends during life.

Deep capillary naevi are less common but more cosmetically disfiguring than superficial lesions. Most occur on the head and neck and are usually unilateral, often appearing in the territory of one or more branches of the trigeminal nerve (Fig. 10.9). They may be small or very extensive.

At birth the colour may vary from pale pink to deep purple, but deep lesions show no tendency to fade. Indeed they may darken with time, and often become progressively thickened. Lumpy, angiomatous nodules may develop.

These lesions are most unattractive, and patients often seek help. The newer types of lasers can produce reasonable results, and there is also a range of cosmetics which can be used as camouflage.

There are three important complications.

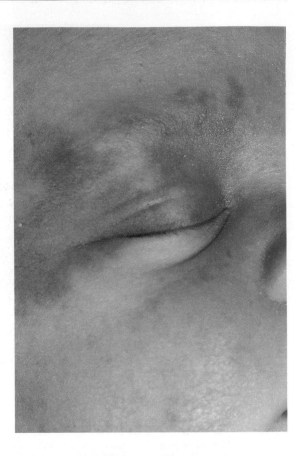

Fig. 10.8 Superficial
capillary naevus.

COMPLICATIONS

- An associated intracranial vascular malformation may result in fits,
  long-tract signs and mental retardation. This is the 'Sturge–Weber
  syndrome'
- Congenital glaucoma may occur in lesions involving the area of the
  ophthalmic division of the trigeminal nerve
- Growth of underlying tissues may be abnormal, resulting in
  hypertrophy of whole limbs—haemangiectatic hypertrophy

If a deep capillary naevus is relatively pale in colour it may be difficult to
distinguish from the superficial type, especially in the neonatal period. It is
therefore important to give a somewhat guarded initial prognosis and
await events.

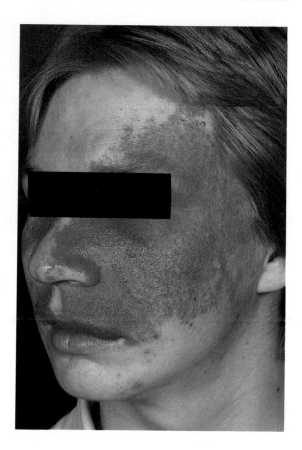

Fig. 10.9 Deep capillary
naevus ('port-wine stain').

Angiomatous naevi

In some accounts these lesions are classified with capillary naevi, whereas in others they are termed 'cavernous'. Most authorities acknowledge that both capillary derived elements and larger, so-called 'cavernous' vascular spaces are usually involved.

STRAWBERRY NAEVUS

Strawberry naevi arise very shortly after birth. They may appear anywhere, but have a predilection for the head and neck and the napkin area (Fig. 10.10). Most are solitary, but occasionally there are more. The lesion grows rapidly to produce a dome-shaped, red–purple extrusion which may bleed if traumatized. The majority reach a maximum size within a few months. They may be large and unsightly.

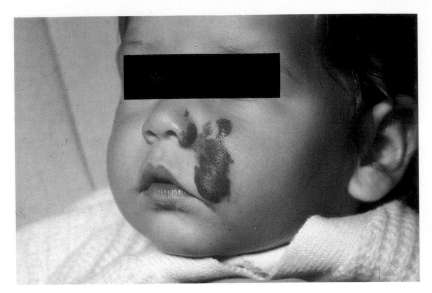

Fig. 10.10 Cavernous haemangioma on the face.

Spontaneous resolution is the norm, sometimes beginning with central necrosis, which can look alarming. As a rule of thumb, 50% have resolved by the age of 5 and 70% by age 7. Some only regress partially, and a few require plastic surgical intervention.

The management, in all but a few, is expectant. It is useful to show parents a series of pictures of previous patients in whom the lesion has resolved

Specific indications for intervention:

1 if breathing or feeding is obstructed;

2 if the tumour occludes an eye—this will lead to blindness (amblyopia);

3 if severe bleeding occurs;

4 if haemorrhage within a large tumour leads to consumption coagulopathy (*Kasabach–Merritt syndrome*);

5 if the tumour remains large and unsightly after the age of 10.

Treatment of complications 1–4 is initially with high-dose prednisolone, which may produce marked shrinkage. If this fails, and in the fifth complication, complex surgical intervention may be required.

RARE ANGIOMATOUS NAEVI

Rarely, infants are born with multiple strawberry naevus-like angiomas of skin and internal organs. This is known as *neonatal angiomatosis* and the prognosis is often poor.

OTHER NAEVI

Naevi may develop from other skin elements, including connective tissue, mast cells and fat. For example, the cutaneous stigmata of tuberous sclerosis are connective tissue naevi (see Chapter 11), and the lesions of urticaria pigmentosa are mast cell naevi.

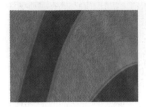

CHAPTER 11

Inherited Disorders

*There is only one more beautiful thing than a fine healthy skin,
and that is a rare skin disease.* (Sir Erasmus Wilson, 1809–84)

A number of skin conditions are known to be inherited. Many are rare, and
will therefore only be mentioned briefly. Several diseases in which genetic
factors play an important part, such as atopic eczema, psoriasis, acne
vulgaris and male pattern balding, are described elsewhere in the book.

THE ICHTHYOSES

The term ichthyosis is derived from the Greek *ichthys*, meaning fish, as the
skin has been likened to fish scales. The ichthyoses are disorders of keratinization in which the skin is extremely dry and scaly (Fig. 11.1). In the
majority of cases the disease is inherited, but occasionally ichthyosis
may be an acquired phenomenon, for example in association with a lymphoma. There are several types of ichthyosis, which have different modes
of inheritance.

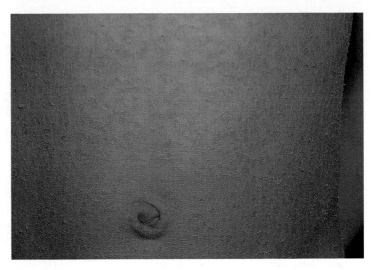

Fig. 11.1 Ichthyosis.

AUTOSOMAL DOMINANT ICHTHYOSIS (ICHTHYOSIS VULGARIS)

This is the commonest, and is often quite mild. The scaling usually appears during early childhood. The skin on the trunk and extensor aspects of the limbs is dry and flaky, but the limb flexures are often spared. Dominant ichthyosis is frequently associated with an atopic constitution.

X-LINKED ICHTHYOSIS

This type of ichthyosis only affects males. The scales are larger and darker than those of dominant ichthyosis, and usually the trunk and limbs are extensively involved, including the flexures. Corneal opacities may occur, but these do not interfere with vision. Affected individuals are deficient in the enzyme steroid sulphatase, and this is thought to be related to the pathogenesis of the ichthyosis, although the precise mechanism is not known.

Both X-linked ichthyosis and autosomal dominant ichthyosis improve during the summer months.

ICHTHYOSIFORM ERYTHRODERMA

A bullous form of this condition is dominantly inherited, and a non-bullous form recessively inherited. In both, the skin is scaly and erythematous, and often has an offensive odour.

TREATMENT

Treatment consists of regular use of emollients and bath oils. Urea-containing creams are also helpful. The more severe types of ichthyosis often require oral retinoid therapy.

COLLODION BABY

This terminology is applied to babies born encased in a transparent rigid membrane (Fig. 11.2). The membrane cracks and peels off after a few days. Some affected babies have an underlying ichthyotic disorder. Collodion babies have increased transepidermal water loss, and it is essential that they are nursed in a high humidity environment and given additional fluids.

PALMOPLANTAR KERATODERMA

Several rare disorders are associated with massive thickening of the horny layer of the palms and soles. The commonest type is dominantly inherited. Many medical texts mention the association of palmoplantar keratoderma (tylosis) with carcinoma of the oesophagus—in fact this is extremely rare.

DARIER'S DISEASE (KERATOSIS FOLLICULARIS)

This is a dominantly inherited abnormality of keratinization which is usually first evident in late childhood or adolescence. The characteristic

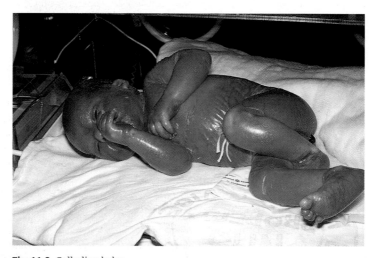

Fig. 11.2 Collodion baby.

lesions of Darier's disease are brown follicular keratotic papules, grouped together over the face and neck, the centre of the chest and back, the axillae and the groins (Fig. 11.3). The nails typically show longitudinal pink or white bands, with V-shaped notches at the free edges. There are usually numerous wart-like lesions on the hands (acrokeratosis verruciformis).

Treatment

Darier's disease responds to treatment with retinoids.

EPIDERMOLYSIS BULLOSA

This group of hereditary blistering diseases is described in Chapter 14.

EHLERS–DANLOS SYNDROME

There are a number of distinct variants of this condition, all of which are associated with abnormalities of collagen, principally defective production.

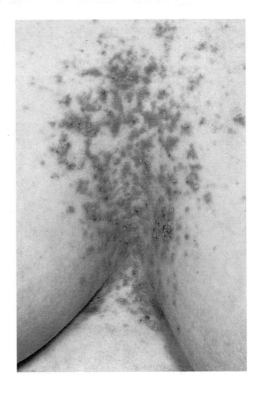

Fig. 11.3 Darier's disease.

The most common are dominantly inherited, but all types of Ehlers–Danlos syndrome are rare. Typical features are skin hyperextensibility and fragility, and joint hypermobility. In certain types there is a risk of rupture of major blood vessels.

TUBEROUS SCLEROSIS (EPILOIA)

This is a dominantly inherited disorder, but many cases are new mutations. There are hamartomatous malformations in the skin and internal organs. Characteristic skin lesions include numerous pink papules on the face (Fig. 11.4) (originally called adenoma sebaceum), which are hematomas of connective tissue and small blood vessels (angiofibromas); the shagreen patch on the back (a connective tissue naevus); periungual fibromas (Fig. 11.5); and hypopigmented macules (ash leaf macules) which are best seen with the aid of Wood's light. The hypopigmented macules are often present at birth, but the facial lesions usually first appear at the age of 5 or 6. Affected individuals may be mentally retarded and suffer from epilepsy. Other features include retinal phakomas, pulmonary and renal hamartomas, and cardiac rhabdomyomas.

NEUROFIBROMATOSIS

Neurofibromatosis (von Recklinghausen's disease) is dominantly inherited, and characterized by multiple café-au-lait patches and numerous

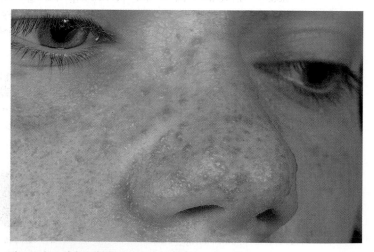

Fig. 11.4 Facial angiofibromata in tuberous sclerosis.

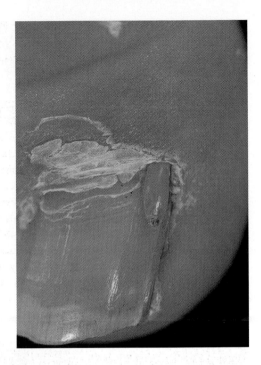

Fig. 11.5 Periungual fibroma in tuberous sclerosis.

neurofibromas (Fig. 11.6). A constant feature is axillary freckling (Crowe's sign). Other associated abnormalities include scoliosis, an increased risk of developing intracranial neoplasms, particularly meningioma, acoustic neuroma and optic nerve glioma, and an increased risk of hypertension associated with phaeochromocytoma or fibromuscular hyperplasia of the renal arteries.

PEUTZ–JEGHERS SYNDROME

In this rare dominantly inherited syndrome there are pigmented macules (lentigines) in the mouth, on the lips, and on the hands and feet, in association with multiple hamartomatous intestinal polyps.

HEREDITARY HAEMORRHAGIC TELANGIECTASIA (OSLER–WEBER–RENDU DISEASE)

This is a rare, dominantly inherited disorder in which multiple telangiectases are present on the face and lips, nasal, buccal and intestinal mucosae.

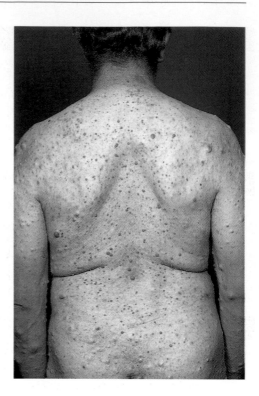

Fig. 11.6 Von Recklinghausen's neurofibromatosis.

Recurrent epistaxes are common, and there is also a risk of gastrointestinal haemorrhage. There is an association with pulmonary and cerebral arteriovenous fistulae.

BASAL CELL NAEVUS SYNDROME (GORLIN'S SYNDROME)

Gorlin's syndrome is a dominantly inherited disorder in which multiple basal cell carcinomata on the face and trunk are associated with characteristic palmar pits, odontogenic keratocysts of the jaw, calcification of the falx cerebri, and skeletal abnormalities.

GARDNER'S SYNDROME

This condition is also dominantly inherited. Affected individuals have multiple epidermoid cysts, osteomas, and large bowel adenomatous polyps which have a high risk of malignant change.

ANHIDROTIC ECTODERMAL DYSPLASIA

This is a rare condition in which eccrine sweat glands are absent or markedly reduced in number, the scalp hair, eyebrows and eyelashes are sparse, and the teeth are widely spaced and conical. The absence of sweating interferes with temperature regulation, and this may lead to hyperthermia in a hot environment. Anhidrotic ectodermal dysplasia is inherited as an X-linked recessive trait.

PSEUDOXANTHOMA ELASTICUM

Four types, two dominant and two recessive, of this disorder of elastin have been described. The skin of the neck and axillae has a lax, 'plucked chicken' appearance of tiny yellowish papules (Fig. 11.7). Retinal angioid streaks, caused by ruptures in Bruch's membrane, are visible on fundoscopy. Abnormal elastic tissue in blood vessels may lead to gastrointestinal haemorrhage.

XERODERMA PIGMENTOSUM

Ultraviolet (UV) damage to epidermal DNA is normally repaired by an enzyme system. In xeroderma pigmentosum, which is recessively inherited, this system is defective, and UV damage is not repaired. This leads to

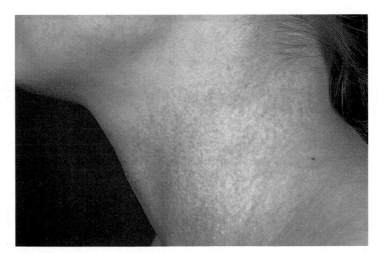

Fig. 11.7 'Plucked chicken' appearance of the skin in pseudoxanthoma elasticum.

the early development of cutaneous neoplasms. Basal cell carcinomas, squamous cell carcinomas and malignant melanomas may all develop in childhood. In some cases there is also gradual neurological deterioration caused by progressive neuronal loss.

ACRODERMATITIS ENTEROPATHICA

In this recessively inherited disorder there is defective absorption of zinc. The condition is usually manifest in early infancy as exudative eczematous lesions around the orifices, and on the hands and feet. Affected infants also suffer from diarrhoea. Acrodermatitis enteropathica can be effectively treated with oral zinc supplements.

ANDERSON–FABRY DISEASE (ANGIOKERATOMA CORPORIS DIFFUSUM)

This condition is the result of an inborn error of glycosphingolipid metabolism. It is inherited in an X-linked recessive manner. Deficiency of the enzyme α-galactosidase leads to deposition of ceramide trihexoside in a number of tissues, including the cardiovascular system, the kidneys, the eyes and peripheral nerves. The skin lesions are tiny vascular angiokeratomas which are usually scattered over the lower trunk, buttocks, genitalia and thighs. Associated features caused by tissue deposition of the lipid include the following.

ANDERSON–FABRY DISEASE

- Premature ischaemic heart disease
- Renal failure
- Severe pain and paraesthesiae in the hands and feet
- Corneal and lens opacities

INCONTINENTIA PIGMENTI

An X-linked dominant disorder, incontinentia pigmenti occurs predominantly in female infants, as it is usually lethal *in utero* in males. Linear bullous lesions are present on the trunk and limbs at birth, or soon thereafter. The bullae are gradually replaced by warty lesions, and these in turn are eventually replaced by streaks and whorls of hyperpigmentation. Incontinentia pigmenti is frequently associated with a variety of ocular, skeletal, dental and central nervous system abnormalities.

CHROMOSOMAL ABNORMALITIES

Some syndromes determined by chromosomal abnormalities may have associated dermatological problems.

ASSOCIATED DERMATOLOGICAL PROBLEMS

- Down's syndrome: increased incidence of alopecia areata
- Turner's syndrome: primary lymphoedema
- Klinefelter's syndrome: premature venous ulceration
- XYY syndrome: premature venous ulceration; prone to develop severe nodulocystic acne

CHAPTER 12

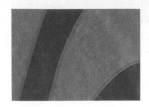

Pigmentary Disorders

> *Bold was her face, and fair, and red of hew.*
>   (Chaucer, *The Wife of Bath*)
> *The complexion of the skin and the colour of the hair correspond to the colour of the moisture which the flesh attracts—white, or red, or black.* (Hippocrates)

INTRODUCTION: NORMAL PIGMENTARY MECHANISMS

Our skin colour is important, and there are many references to it in prose and poetry. We all note skin colour in our initial assessment of someone, and skin colour has been used to justify all manner of injustices. Any departure from the perceived norm can have serious psychological effects, and some practical implications.

A number of factors give rise to our skin colour:

SKIN COLOUR FACTORS

- Haemoglobin
- Exogenous pigments in or on the skin surface
- Endogenously produced pigments (e.g. bilirubin)
- Melanin and phaeomelanin

The last two are the most important in dictating our basic skin colour

Normal pigmentary mechanisms have already been outlined in Chapter 1. Humans have a rather dull range of natural colours when compared with peacocks or parrots: we normally produce only shades of brown and red. Brown is due to melanin, the intensity varying from almost white (no melanin) to virtually jet-black (a large amount). This is determined by genetics in an autosomal dominant manner.

Red is a bonus; only some people are able to produce 'phaeomelanin'. Red is much commoner in some races (e.g. Celts) than in others (e.g. Chinese).

Most of human skin pigment is within keratinocytes, having been manufactured in melanocytes and transferred in 'melanosomes'. There are racial differences in production, distribution and degradation of melanosomes, but not in the number of melanocytes (see Chapter 1). There are, however, important genetic differences in the ability to respond to ultraviolet radiation, conventionally called 'skin types'.

SKIN TYPES

- Type I—always burns, never tans
- Type II—burns easily, tans poorly
- Type III—burns occasionally, tans easily
- Type IV—never burns, tans easily
- Type V—genetically brown (e.g. Indian) or Mongoloid
- Type VI—genetically black (Congoid or Negroid)

The first response to UV radiation is an increased distribution of melanosomes. This rapidly increases basal layer pigmentation—the sun tan. If stimulation is quickly withdrawn, as typically happens after 2 weeks in the Mediterranean, the tan fades rapidly and peels off with normal epidermal turnover. If exposure is prolonged, melanin *production* is stepped up more permanently. Tanning represents the skin's efforts to offer protection from the harmful effects of UV radiation, such as premature ageing and cancers.

We shall now look at states in which these pigmentary mechanisms appear to be abnormal, leading to decreased (hypo-) or increased (hyper-) pigmentation.

HYPOPIGMENTATION

Among the most important causes of hypopigmentation are:

HYPOPIGMENTATION CAUSES

Congenital
- Albinism
- Phenylketonuria
- Tuberous sclerosis
- Hypochromic naevi

Acquired
- Vitiligo
- Sutton's halo naevi
- Tuberculoid leprosy
- Pityriasis (tinea) versicolor
- Pityriasis alba
- Lichen sclerosus et atrophicus
- Drugs and chemicals:
  occupational leucoderma
  self-inflicted/iatrogenic
- Post-inflammatory hypopigmentation

Congenital

Some individuals are born with generalized or localized defects in the pigmentary system.

Albinism and *phenylketonuria* are due to defects in melanin production. In albinos, the enzyme tyrosinase may be *absent* (tyrosinase-negative albinism) leading to generalized white skin and hair, and red eyes (the iris is also depigmented). Vision is usually markedly impaired, with nystagmus.

In tyrosinase-positive albinism (where the enzyme tyrosinase is *defective*), the clinical picture is not as severe, and colour may gradually darken with age. However, skin cancers are much more common in both forms. Albinism also illustrates the importance of colour: in some societies albinos are rejected and despised, in others they are revered as something wonderful.

The biochemical defect in phenylketonuria results in a reduced level of tyrosine, the precursor of melanin, and increased amounts of phenylalanine (which inhibits tyrosinase). There is a generalized reduction in pigmentation of the skin, hair and eyes.

One of the cardinal signs of *tuberous sclerosis (epiloia)* is hypopigmented macules. These are often lanceolate (ash-leaf shaped), but may assume bizarre shapes. They are often present before other external markers. Any infant who presents with fits should be examined for such lesions, and they are easier to see under Wood's light (see Chapter 2). Occasionally, identical localized pale areas are seen without any other abnormality, when they are termed *hypochromic naevi*.

Acquired

Acquired hypopigmentation is common and, in darker skin, may have a particular stigma. This is partly because the cosmetic appearance of patchy hypopigmentation is much worse, but also because white patches are inextricably linked in some cultures with leprosy. Historically all white patches were probably classified as leprosy: Naaman (who was cured of 'leprosy' after bathing in the Jordan [2 Kings 5:1–14]) probably had vitiligo (see below).

Vitiligo is the most important cause of patches of pale skin. The skin in vitiligo becomes *de*pigmented and not hypopigmented, although during *progression* this is not always complete.

Characteristically there is complete loss of pigment from otherwise entirely normal skin (Fig. 12.1). Patches may be small, but commonly become quite large, often with irregular outlines. Depigmentation may spread to involve wide areas of the body. Although vitiligo can occur anywhere, it is often strikingly symmetrical, involving the hands, perioral and periocular skin.

The pathophysiology is poorly understood. In early patches melanocytes are still present, but produce no melanin. Later, melanocytes disappear completely, except deep around hair follicles. Vitiligo may be an

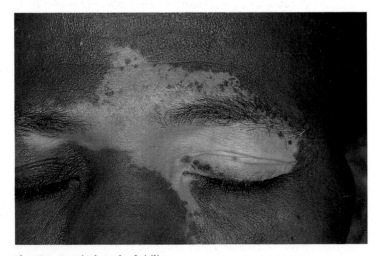

Fig. 12.1 A typical patch of vitiligo.

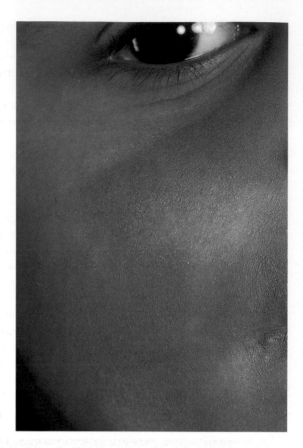

Fig. 12.2 Pityriasis alba on the cheek.

autoimmune process: there is an increase in organ-specific autoantibodies (as in alopecia areata, with which vitiligo is also linked).

Treatment is generally unsatisfactory. Topical steroids have their advocates, and PUVA helps some. Cosmetic camouflage may be helpful. Sun-screens should be used in the summer, because vitiliginous areas will not tan.

In some patients, particularly children, areas may repigment spontaneously. This is less common in adults and in long-standing areas. Repigmentation, when it does happen, often begins with small dots coinciding with hair follicles.

A similar appearance occurs in *Sutton's halo naevus* (see Chapter 10).

Some of the stigma associated with hypopigmentation is because *tuberculoid leprosy* is another cause. The (usually solitary) patch of hypopigmented skin also exhibits diminished sensation. Pale patches may also be seen in the very earliest stages: so-called 'indeterminate' leprosy.

The organism which causes *pityriasis versicolor* (see Chapter 4) produces a chemical (azelaic acid) which results in hypopigmentation. The effect is most noticeable after sun exposure.

Pityriasis alba is a very common cause of hypopigmentation in children, especially in darker skins. Pale patches with a slightly scaly surface appear on the face and upper arms (Fig. 12.2). The underlying process is a low-grade eczema which usually responds (albeit slowly) to moisturizers, but may require mild topical steroids. The tendency appears to clear at puberty.

Lichen sclerosus et atrophicus (see Chapter 15) usually affects the genitalia. On other sites it is sometimes called 'white spot disease'.

Drugs and chemicals may cause loss of skin pigment. These may be encountered at work, but a more common source is skin lightening creams, sold in chemists, especially in areas with Afro-Caribbean populations. The active ingredient is generally hydroquinone, which can be used therapeutically (see below).

Many inflammatory skin disorders may produce secondary or *post-inflammatory* hypopigmentation. This is due to a disturbance in the integrity of the epidermis and its melanin production system, which normally recovers. Eczema and psoriasis often leave hypopigmentation when they resolve. However, inflammation can destroy melanocytes altogether, as occurs in scars, after burns, and in areas treated with cryotherapy (it is the basis of 'freeze-branding').

HYPERPIGMENTATION

As with hypopigmentation, there are many causes of increased skin pigmentation, including excessive production of melanin, or the deposition in the skin of several other pigments, such as β-carotene, bilirubin, drugs and metals: these causes are as follows.

CAUSES OF HYPERPIGMENTATION

Congenital
- Neurofibromatosis
- Peutz-Jeghers syndrome
- LEOPARD syndrome
- Incontinentia pigmenti

Continued on p. 172

CAUSES OF HYPERPIGMENTATION (Continued)

Acquired
- Urticaria pigmentosa
- Addison's disease
- Renal failure
- Haemochromatosis
- Liver disease
- Carotenaemia:
    idiopathic
    myxoedema
    pernicious anaemia
- Acanthosis nigricans
- Chloasma
- Drugs and chemicals
- Post-inflammatory hyperpigmentation

Congenital

Hyperpigmentation is prominent in *neurofibromatosis*, in which café-au-lait marks (Fig. 12.3) and axillary freckling are common. Speckled lentiginous pigmentation is seen around the mouth and on the hands in the *Peutz–Jeghers syndrome*, and similar but more widespread lentigines may accompany a number of congenital defects in the *'LEOPARD' syndrome*.

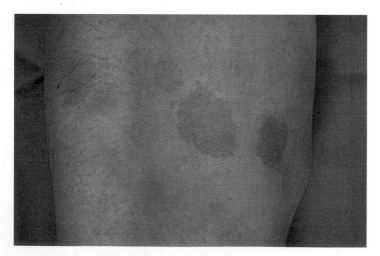

Fig. 12.3 Café-au-lait patches in neurofibromatosis.

Incontinentia pigmenti is a rare congenital disorder which causes hyperpigmentation in a whorled pattern, often with blisters and hyperkeratotic lesions, and other congenital abnormalities.

Acquired

Urticaria pigmentosa is most common in children, but may affect adults. There is a widespread eruption of indistinct brown marks which urticate if rubbed. The disorder is due to abnormal numbers of dermal mast cells.

Chloasma, or melasma, is commoner in women than men. A characteristic pattern of hyperpigmentation develops on the forehead, cheeks and chin (Fig. 12.4). It is exaggerated by sunlight. Provoking factors include pregnancy and the oral contraceptive pill, but chloasma may occur spontaneously. Treatment is difficult. Avoidance of precipitating factors (especially sunlight and oestrogens) may help. Topical hydroquinone preparations are sometimes used.

Various drugs and chemicals can cause cutaneous hyperpigmentation (see Chapter 21).

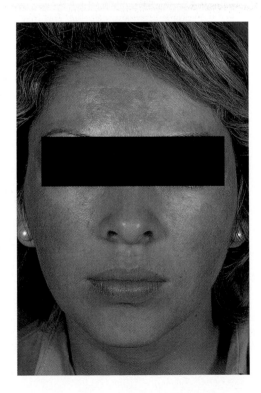

Fig. 12.4 Typical chloasma.

In *post-inflammatory* hyperpigmentation disruption of the lower layers of the epidermis results in deposition of melanin granules in the dermis (pigmentary incontinence). Many skin disorders do this, particularly in pigmented skin, but lichen planus is particularly troublesome. There is no useful treatment, but the pigmentation gradually fades with time.

Hyperpigmentation is an important physical sign in several systemic diseases.

1 *Addison's disease*—the changes are most marked in the skin creases, in scratch marks, and the gums.

2 *Renal failure*—may cause a muddy-brown skin colour.

3 *Haemochromatosis*—causes a deep golden-brown hue, diabetes and liver disease.

4 *Some chronic liver diseases*—result in deep pigmentation.

β-*Carotene* (a yellow pigment) accumulates harmlessly in the skin in some normal individuals who ingest large amounts of carrots and orange juice (rich sources). The colour is most marked on the palms and soles. Similar deposition is seen in some patients with myxoedema and pernicious anaemia.

Another important, although rare, cause of acquired hyperpigmentation is *acanthosis nigricans*. This may or may not be associated with a systemic disease (see Chapter 19).

CHAPTER 13

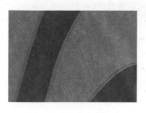

Disorders
of the Hair
and Nails

If a woman have long hair, it is a glory to her.
St Paul (1 Corinthians, 11:15).
The hair takes root in the head at the same time as the nails grow.
(Hippocrates)

INTRODUCTION

Hippocrates (see above) clearly knew that hair and nails were intimately connected, but there are many conditions which affect one or the other alone. We will deal first with abnormalities of hair and then nail disorders, but there will inevitably be some overlap.

Abnormalities of hair and nails may be the result of:

1 local factors;
2 generalized skin disease;
3 systemic disease.

HAIR ABNORMALITIES

Hair is important psychologically. Disturbances in growth or physical characteristics, even of minor degree, may be very distressing: only Kojak really liked being bald! Remember that the distress caused is not necessarily proportionate to the severity apparent to an observer.

Patients present with three main hair abnormalities:

1 changes in physical properties, such as colour or texture;
2 thinning or loss of hair;
3 excessive hair growth, including growth in abnormal sites.

Changes in physical properties of scalp hair

Common physical changes which are seen in hair are as follows.

PHYSICAL CHANGES TO HAIR

Pigmentation
- Genetic diseases, e.g. albinism, phenylketonuria
- Premature greying:
  physiological
  pathological, e.g. pernicious anaemia
- Ageing
- Vitiligo
- Alopecia areata

Textural abnormalities
- Brittleness
- Coarseness
- Curliness

CHANGE IN COLOUR

Greying of the hair, whether premature or not, is permanent, and this usually applies to the white hair in scalp vitiligo. Regrowing hair in alopecia areata (see below) is often white initially, but usually repigments later.

TEXTURAL ABNORMALITIES

Brittleness or coarseness may accompany hair thinning in hypothyroidism and in iron deficiency (see below). Hair may also become 'lack-lustre' from certain hairdressing techniques ('back-combing', bleaching and drying). In men, hair may become curly in the early stages of androgenetic alopecia (see below).

Scalp hair loss

Abnormal scalp hair loss is a feature of some congenital disorders.

CONGENITAL DISORDERS

- Ectodermal dysplasias
- Premature ageing syndromes
- Monilethrix
- Pili torti
- Marie–Unna alopecia

Continued on p. 177

CONGENITAL DISORDERS (Continued)

- Disorders of amino acid metabolism
- Scalp naevi (especially epithelial or organoid)
- Aplasia cutis

Very few of these conditions are amenable to treatment, but they require careful assessment, often including microscopic examination of hair shafts.

ACQUIRED DISORDERS

Patients most commonly seek advice about hair loss when it is from the scalp, although other areas may be affected. The most effective approach to the diagnosis of acquired scalp hair loss is to consider:

1 whether the changes are diffuse or circumscribed, and
2 to assess the state of the scalp skin.

Such an approach, together with some knowledge of the disorders mentioned below leads to a working classification.

ACQUIRED CAUSES OF SCALP HAIR LOSS

Diffuse hair loss with normal scalp skin
- Telogen effluvium
- Thyroid disease
- Iron deficiency
- Drugs
- Systemic lupus erythematosus
- Secondary syphilis
- Alopecia totalis

Androgenetic alopecia

Circumscribed hair loss with normal scalp skin
- Alopecia areata
- Traction
- Trichotillomania
- Tinea capitis (Chapter 4)

Continued on p. 178

ACQUIRED CAUSES OF SCALP HAIR LOSS (*Continued*)

Hair loss with abnormal scalp skin

Without scarring
- Severe psoriasis or seborrhoeic dermatitis
- Tinea capitis (Chapter 4)

With scarring
- Discoid lupus erythematosus
- Lichen planus
- Pseudopelade
- Cicatricial pemphigoid
- Trigeminal trophic syndrome
- Lupus vulgaris

Telogen effluvium is often triggered by major illness, operations, accidents or other stress. The growth of many hairs suddenly stops and they rapidly enter the resting or 'telogen' phase, and fall out about 3 months later. Therefore, ask whether there has been any major upset in the appropriate period. Pull gently on hairs on the crown or sides, and several will come out easily. With a hand lens the bulb looks much smaller than normal. Telogen effluvium settles spontaneously, but can unmask androgenetic alopecia (see below), and some patients find their hair never returns completely to normal.

Appropriate tests will exclude the important systemic diseases listed above, and correct treatment may restore hair growth.

Many drugs can induce hair loss.

DRUGS INDUCING HAIR LOSS

- Cytotoxic agents
- Anti-thyroid agents, especially thiouracil
- Anticoagulants
- Vitamin A analogues
- Thallium

All of these processes can be confused with alopecia areata (see below) when the latter is widespread and rapidly progressive.

Androgenetic alopecia (or common balding) occurs in both men and women. It is due to the effects of androgens in genetically susceptible individuals.

In men, the process may begin at any age after puberty, but it is much more common from the 30s onwards. Eighty per cent show some hair loss by age 70. Hair is usually lost first at the temples and/or on the crown, but there may be complete hair loss, sparing a parieto-occipital rim. Terminal hairs become progressively finer and smaller, until only a few vellus hairs remain. The extent and pace of this varies widely.

In women the process is slower and less severe, but causes much distress. Up to half of all women have mild hair loss on the vertex by age 50, and in some more severe thinning occurs. There may be accompanying hirsutism (see below).

Until recently there was no known treatment, but there is some evidence that early use of topical minoxidil may help.

CIRCUMSCRIBED HAIR LOSS WITH NORMAL SCALP SKIN

Alopecia areata

The cause of this disorder is unknown but it is strongly suspected that it is an autoimmune process. Organ-specific autoantibodies (to thyroid, adrenal or gastric parietal cells) are often found in the patients' sera.

History: one or more areas of baldness suddenly appear on the scalp, in the eyebrows, beard, or elsewhere. It is most common in childhood or early adult life, although periodic recurrences throughout life may occur, and it can begin much later.

Examination: patches are typically round or oval (Fig. 13.1); the skin usually appears completely normal, although there may be mild erythema; a number of areas may develop next to each other, giving rise to a moth-eaten appearance; close examination of the edge of a patch of alopecia areata reveals the pathognomonic feature—'exclamation mark hairs'—\short hairs which taper towards their bases (Fig. 13.2).

Prognosis: most patches regrow after a few weeks, although further episodes can occur; initial hair growth may be white; occasionally, the process continues to spread and may become permanent—if this state involves the whole scalp it is termed *alopecia totalis* and if the whole body is affected, the name *alopecia universalis* is applied. The nails may be affected in severe cases (see below).

Treatment: this is difficult, but intralesional steroids may help, and topical sensitizers such as dinitrochlorobenzene and diphencyprone are also used.

Chronic traction can also cause circumscribed alopecia, often around scalp margins (Fig. 13.3). It is commonly seen in young girls with tight 'pony

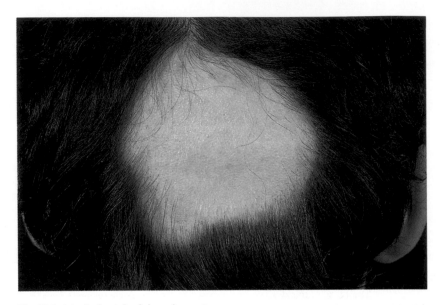

Fig. 13.1 A typical patch of alopecia areata.

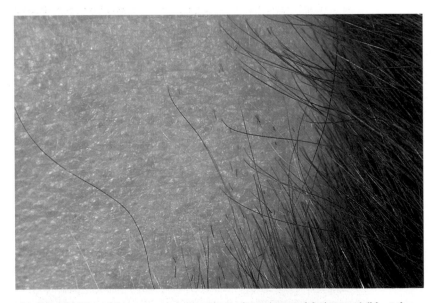

Fig. 13.2 The edge of the area seen in Fig. 13.1. Exclamation mark hairs are visible at the margin.

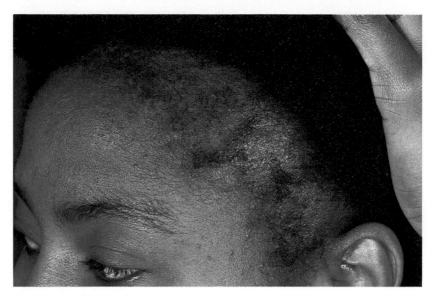

Fig. 13.3 Traction alopecia.

tails', Sikh boys and Afro-Caribbean children whose hair is dressed in multiple little 'pigtails'.

In *trichotillomania*, hair is pulled, twisted or rubbed out, and affected site(s) are covered in a stubble of broken hairs. There may be psychological factors (see Chapter 20).

HAIR LOSS WITH ABNORMAL SCALP SKIN

Psoriasis, seborrhoeic dermatitis and other inflammatory processes can cause temporary hair loss. Another important cause of temporary hair loss with scalp inflammation is tinea capitis (see Chapter 4).

In some conditions fibrosis accompanies the inflammation, and this may result in permanent damage to hair follicles, and obvious loss of tissue or atrophy. This is known as *scarring* or *cicatricial* alopecia.

Examination of the rest of the skin may provide clues to the aetiology of the alopecia.

CAUSES OF CICATRICIAL ALOPECIA

Discoid lupus erythematosus
- Prominent plugging of the hair follicles
- Look for lesions on the face

Continued on p. 182

CAUSES OF CICATRICIAL ALOPECIA
(Continued)

Lichen planus
- May accompany lichen planus elsewhere
- Nail involvement is common (see Chapter 15)

Cicatricial pemphigoid
- Alopecia follows blistering

Lupus vulgaris (cutaneous TB)
- Especially in international residents

Trigeminal trophic syndrome
- May follow herpes zoster because of hypoaesthesia and chronic trauma

Pseudopelade
- Small patches of scarring alopecia without distinguishing features

In most of these conditions a biopsy is essential. In cases where lupus erythematosus or cicatricial pemphigoid are suspected, immunofluorescence should also be performed.

GENERALIZED HAIR LOSS

Generalized hair loss is rare, but may accompany endocrine disturbances, especially *hypothyroidism* or *hypopituitarism*. Drugs, particularly cytotoxics, may induce widespread alopecia. As has been mentioned, alopecia areata may lead to complete hair loss—*alopecia universalis*.

Excessive hair and hair in abnormal sites

HIRSUTISM

This term is applied to excessive growth of hair in a female, distributed in a male secondary sexual pattern.

CAUSES OF HIRSUTISM

- Mild hirsutism is quite common in elderly women
- It may be a genetic trait in younger females, when the changes may also accompany a general reduction in scalp hair (see androgenetic alopecia above)
- Minor endocrine disturbances, especially polycystic ovary syndrome
- Drugs with androgenic activity
- Virilizing tumours

A search for more serious causes is indicated if the changes are of rapid onset.

Treatment includes shaving, waxing and electrolysis. The anti-androgen cyproterone acetate may help.

HYPERTRICHOSIS

Excessive hair growth in a non-sexual distribution may occur in both sexes. There are several causes:

CAUSES OF HYPERTRICHOSIS

- Congenital generalized: e.g. Cornelia de Lange syndrome
- Congenital localized: e.g. 'faun-tail' in spina bifida occulta
- Drugs such as:
  minoxidil (now used for baldness — see above)
  cyclosporin
  hydantoins
  systemic steroids
- Anorexia nervosa
- Cachexia
- Porphyria cutanea tarda: associated with scarring and milia
- Pretibial myxoedema: overlying plaques

NAIL ABNORMALITIES

Nail changes may be non-specific, or characteristic of specific processes. They may occur in isolation, but the nails are abnormal in several disorders:

DISORDERS WITH ABNORMAL NAILS

Congenital
- Especially disorders of keratinization, e.g. Darier's disease
- Ectodermal dysplasias
- Due to scarring, e.g. dystrophic epidermolysis bullosa

Acquired
- Psoriasis
- Eczema/dermatitis
- Lichen planus
- Alopecia areata/totalis
- Fungal infections

COMMON NAIL ABNORMALITIES

Brittleness
- Increases with age
- Seen in iron deficiency (see also koilonychia) and thyroid disease

Roughness (trachyonychia)
- Common and often non-specific
- May result from widespread pitting (see below)

Beau's lines
- Horizontal grooves due to major illness

Pits
- Classical feature of psoriasis
- Severe alopecia areata (smaller, more evenly distributed)
- Eczema/dermatitis (coarse dents and irregular pits)

Onycholysis (Fig. 13.4)
- Lifting of nail plate off nail bed
- Causes:
  psoriasis
  fungal infection (see Chapter 14)
  thyrotoxicosis
  space-occupying lesion (e.g. exostosis or tumour)
- May be no other identifiable abnormality present

Clubbing
- Sign of pulmonary, liver or thyroid disease; may be familial

Discolouration
- White marks—common normal variant
- White nails—underlying cirrhosis
- Pale—anaemia
- Half red/half pale—renal disease
- Sulphur yellow—fungal infection
- Uniform yellow—'yellow nail syndrome' (+ bronchiectasis and lymphoedema)
- Green–blue—*Pseudomonas* infection
- Brown–black —melanoma, haematoma
- Linear brown—naevus

Koilonychia
- Nails with a concave upper surface (spoon-shaped)
- Causes:

Continued on p. 185

COMMON NAIL ABNORMALITIES (Continued)

iron deficiency
inherited

Washboard nails
- Habitual picking of nail fold leads to surface ridging

Onychogryphosis
- Grossly thickened, distorted nails (Fig. 13.5) often due to neglect

'Pterygium'
- Damage leads to epithelium encroaching on nail surface
- Cause—lichen planus

Loss of nails
- Causes:
  pterygium
  scarring, e.g. Stevens—Johnson syndrome
  severe inflammation, e.g. pustular psoriasis
  malignant tumours

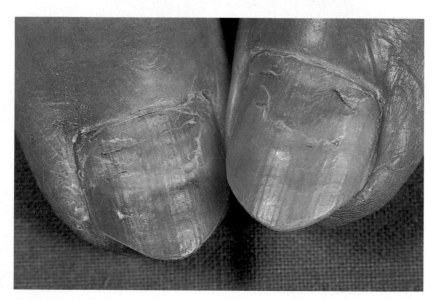

Fig. 13.4 Onycholysis of the nails in a woman with no other relevant findings.

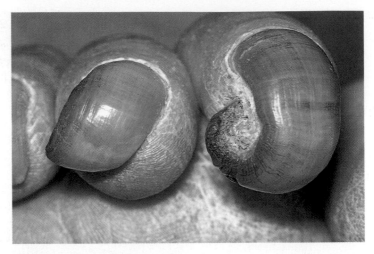

Fig. 13.5 Onychogryphosis.

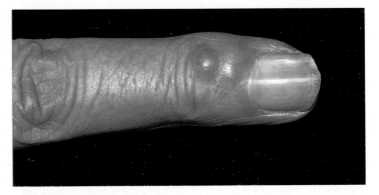

Fig. 13.6 Myxoid cyst of the finger.

Common disorders of the paronychium

Patients may also complain of disorders of the area around the nail—the paronychium.

PARONYCHIA

There are two common forms, acute and chronic. In acute paronychia, an abscess in the nail fold forms, points and discharges. It is nearly always staphylococcal. Chronic paronychia is discussed in Chapter 4.

INGROWING NAILS

Overcurved nails (especially on big toes) dig into the lateral nail fold leading to chronic inflammation and overproduction of granulation tissue. Sometimes this can be prevented by trimming nails straight, but surgical intervention is often required.

PERIUNGUAL WARTS

Warts are discussed in Chapter 3. Periungual warts are unsightly and are often extremely difficult to eradicate.

MYXOID CYST

Small cystic swellings may appear on the proximal nail fold (Fig. 13.6). The nail may develop a linear depression. Clear gelatinous fluid can be expressed, if the surface is breached. These cysts are commoner in the middle-aged and elderly and are due to a degenerative process. Treatment is difficult.

CHAPTER 14

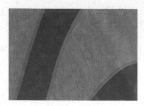

Bullous Disorders

All that blisters is not pemphigus (Graham-Brown and Burns, 1990)

CAUSES

The skin has a limited repertoire of changes, but few are more dramatic than an eruption of blisters or bullae. There are many causes.

CAUSES OF BULLAE

Physical
- Cold, heat, friction, oedema

Infections (see Chapters 3 and 4)

Bacterial
- Impetigo

Viral
- Chickenpox
- Herpes zoster
- Herpes simplex
- Smallpox and vaccinia
- Hand, foot and mouth disease

Fungal
- Tinea pedis with pompholyx

Arthropods (see Chapter 5)
- Insect bites

Continued on p. 189

CAUSES OF BULLAE (Continued)

Drugs (see also Chapter 21)
- Barbiturates, sulphonamides, iodides, frusemide, nalidixic acid (light-induced)
- Drug-induced pemphigus and pemphigoid
- Fixed drug eruptions

Skin disorders

Congenital
- Epidermolysis bullosa

Acquired
Bullae are a major feature in:
- Pemphigus
- Bullous pemphigoid
- Cicatricial pemphigoid
- Dermatitis herpetiformis
- 'Linear IgA disease'
- Epidermolysis bullosa acquisita
- Toxic epidermal necrolysis
- Subcorneal pustular dermatosis

Bullae may occur in:
- Erythema multiforme (Stevens–Johnson syndrome)
- Eczema (including pompholyx)
- Lichen planus
- Psoriasis (pustular)
- Vasculitis

Metabolic disease
- Porphyria cutanea tarda, diabetes mellitus

This is a fairly comprehensive differential diagnostic list for further reading.

Some, such as impetigo and the viral causes, are mentioned elsewhere. This chapter is concerned with the most important of the remaining causes of blistering.

Physical causes of bullae

Burns may result from cold, heat or chemical injury and are common causes of blisters, as is extreme friction (e.g. the feet of vigorous squash players or joggers). Severe, acute oedema of the lower legs in congestive cardiac failure may also produce tense bullae.

Arthropods

Remember that insect bites very commonly present as tense bullae (see Chapter 5). In the UK, this is most common in late summer and early autumn (fall).

Drugs

Several drugs cause blistering (see above). Blisters caused by nalidixic acid occur on the lower legs following sun exposure. Fixed drug eruptions may blister; they are discussed in Chapter 21.

Skin disorders

Primary skin disorders giving rise to bullae may be congenital or acquired. In some, bullae are an important or integral part of the clinical presentation. In others, blisters may occur but are not the most prominent or constant feature, and the reader should consult the appropriate chapter for further information.

CONGENITAL

Epidermolysis bullosa

Although very rare, this is an important group of disorders. Babies are born with fragile skin which blisters on contact, due to splits within the skin which may occur at different levels. There are several variants; all are unpleasant and some are fatal.

Diagnosis requires electron microscopy to determine the level of the blister. However, the differential diagnosis of blistering in a neonate must also include a number of other disorders:

1 impetigo (pemphigus neonatorum);
2 staphylococcal scalded skin syndrome (see below);
3 incontinentia pigmenti (Chapter 11).

ACQUIRED

Pemphigus

The cardinal processes in all forms of pemphigus are:
1 a split within the epidermis;
2 loss of adhesion of epidermal cells ('acantholysis').

These changes may be just above the basal layer (pemphigus vulgaris; Fig. 14.1) or higher in the epidermis (pemphigus foliaceous; Fig. 14.2).

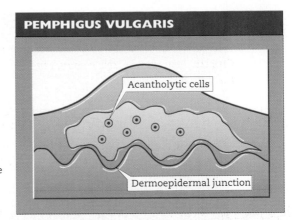

Fig. 14.1 Pemphigus vulgaris: split just above the basal layer, with overlying acantholysis of epidermal cells.

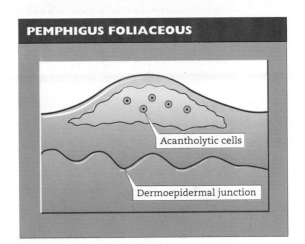

Fig. 14.2 Pemphigus foliaceous: similar changes to Fig. 14.1 but higher in the epidermis.

The commonest variant is *pemphigus vulgaris*, which presents with flaccid blisters and erosions (Fig. 14.3). These may be anywhere, but in over 50% of patients the disorder involves the mouth (Fig. 14.4), causing erosions. Perineal lesions are also common. The blisters rupture easily and the resulting erosions heal very slowly, if at all. A highly characteristic feature is the *Nikolsky sign*: skin at the edge of a blister slides off when pushed by a finger or picked up with forceps. This sign is virtually pathognomonic as it is only seen in pemphigus and toxic epidermal necrolysis (see below). *Pemphigus vegetans* is a variant of pemphigus vulgaris in which vegetating masses occur, especially in the flexures.

Pemphigus foliaceous does not always present with obvious blisters, because they are even more fragile than in pemphigus vulgaris. In the early

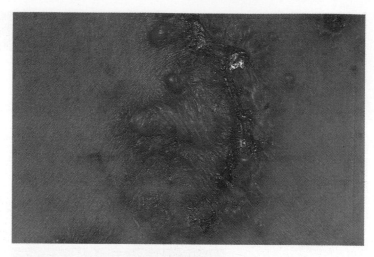

Fig. 14.3 Pemphigus vulgaris: flaccid blisters and erosions.

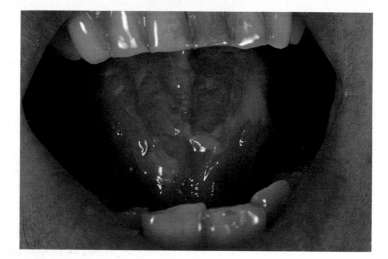

Fig. 14.4 Pemphigus: oral erosions.

stages there may only be non-specific scaly areas, and scalp and face involvement can closely simulate seborrhoeic eczema. One variant known as *pemphigus erythematosus* remains localized to the face, and may be confused with lupus erythematosus.

Investigations

The investigations of all forms of pemphigus are the same:

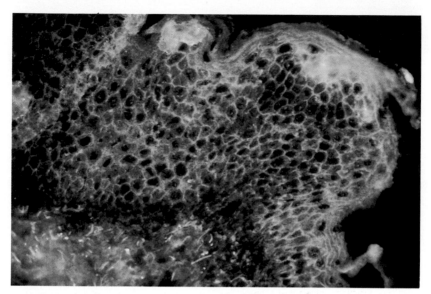

Fig. 14.5 Pemphigus: direct immunofluorescence. IgG is found around epidermal cells.

1 biopsies from involved skin, preserving a blister intact if possible, for histopathology;

2 perilesional tissue for direct immunofluorescence;

3 serum for indirect immunofluorescence.

The immunopathology of pemphigus vulgaris and foliaceous is identical:

1 bright staining around epidermal cells with antibodies directed against immunoglobulin G (IgG) and C3 (Fig. 14.5);

2 circulating anti-epithelial antibody (in the majority of patients).

Treatment

Treatment of pemphigus must be vigorous. Before systemic cortico-steroids were available most patients died, often after a long and debilitating illness.

High doses of prednisolone (60–120 mg daily) are used. The dose is gradually reduced when new blistering has ceased (usually in about 4–6 weeks). Immunosuppressive agents such as azathioprine, chlorambucil, cyclophosphamide or methotrexate may be added as steroid-sparing agents.

Good nursing and metabolic management are crucial because pemphigus patients may be systemically ill. Widespread erosions cause loss of protein and fluid, and secondary infection is common. If the

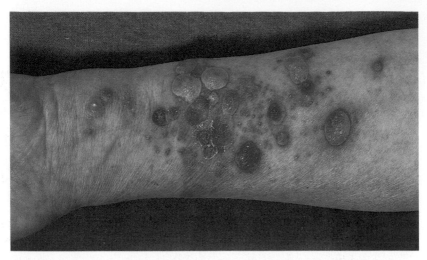

Fig. 14.6 Bullous pemphigoid: tense blisters with an erythematous base arising on a typical site.

mouth is severely involved, patients cannot eat and may be severely catabolic.

Bullous pemphigoid and cicatricial pemphigoid

Bullous pemphigoid is much commoner than pemphigus. More than 80% of patients are over 60 years of age.

Bullae are the most characteristic feature, but they are not always present initially: the process may begin with a non-specific phase known as 'pre-pemphigoid', characterized by intense irritation and well-defined, slightly elevated, erythematous areas.

The bullae, which are usually numerous, are tense and dome-shaped, and may be blood-filled (Fig. 14.6). They vary from a few millimetres to several centimetres in diameter. They often arise on urticated erythema as described above, but are also seen on normal skin. Although the lesions may appear anywhere, there is a marked predilection for the limbs. Oral involvement occurs in about 30%. When blisters burst, healing is usually rapid. Some blisters do not burst, and the fluid is simply reabsorbed. Scarring is not normally seen.

There is, however, a distinctive variant in which marked scarring results, known as *cicatricial* pemphigoid. This condition has a predilection for oral, conjunctival and genital epithelium.

The diagnosis in both forms of pemphigoid requires:

1 a biopsy for histopathology;

2 a biopsy for immunofluorescence;

3 serum for indirect immunofluorescence (less valuable).

The pathological findings are as follows:

PATHOLOGICAL FINDINGS

- A sub-epidermal blister (Fig. 14.7)
- A linear band of IgG and C3 at the basement membrane zone (Fig. 14.8)
- A circulating IgG antibody to basement membrane in 70% of patients with bullous pemphigoid
- No circulating antibody in cicatricial pemphigoid

Treatment

Both variants require treatment with systemic steroids, in moderate doses, usually with immunosuppressives such as azathioprine or chlorambucil.

Bullous pemphigoid usually responds rapidly, and maintenance therapy with small doses is usually possible. The condition appears to be self-limiting in some. Cicatricial pemphigoid is much less responsive.

Dermatitis herpetiformis and linear IgA disease

Dermatitis herpetiformis is uncommon. Its importance lies in its ability to cause severe itching, and its association with a gluten-sensitive enteropathy.

Clinically, the cardinal feature is pruritus, associated with grouped erythematous papules and vesicles. The sites of predilection are the elbows (Fig. 14.9) and extensor surfaces of the forearms, knees and shins, buttocks, shoulders and scalp.

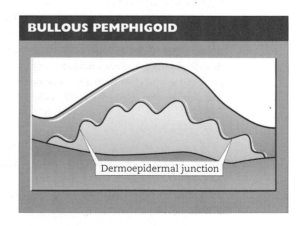

BULLOUS PEMPHIGOID

Dermoepidermal junction

Fig. 14.7 Bullous pemphigoid: the split is sub-epidermal.

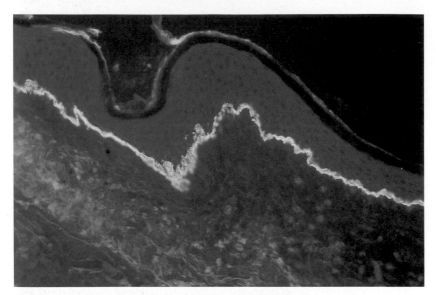

Fig. 14.8 Bullous pemphigoid: direct immunofluorescence. IgG at the basement membrane zone.

The intense itching may result in excoriations, secondary eczematization and lichenification. It is often difficult to find intact vesicles or bullae because of this.

Dermatitis herpetiformis should be considered in any patient who has atypical eczema or pruritus localized to the areas mentioned above.

The diagnosis requires:

1 a biopsy of a blister or, preferably, a *new pink papule* for histopathology;
2 a biopsy of *normal skin* for immunofluorescence;
3 a jejunal biopsy.

The main pathological findings are as follows.

PATHOLOGICAL FINDINGS

- A sub-epidermal blister which is indistinguishable, when fully formed and intact, from that seen in bullous pemphigoid
- *However*, in very early, pre-vesicular lesions (hence the pink papule), or at the edge of a vesicle, there are small neutrophil 'microabscesses' in dermal papillary tips (Fig. 14.10). These are pathognomonic
- *Granular* IgA in the dermal papillary tips on immunofluorescence (Fig. 14.11)
- There are no circulating antibodies
- Gut changes range from an increase in lymphocyte numbers to various grades of villous atrophy

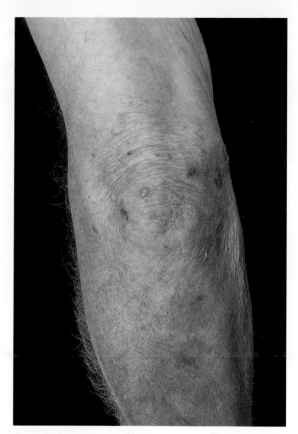

Fig. 14.9 Dermatitis herpetiformis: the elbow is a typical site.

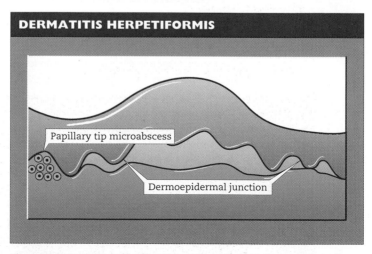

Fig. 14.10 Dermatitis herpetiformis: papillary tip microabscesses as well as a sub-epidermal blister.

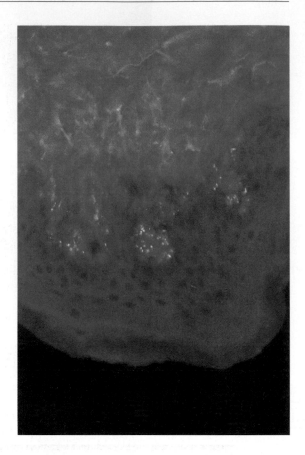

Fig. 14.11 Dermatitis herpetiformis: immunofluorescence of normal skin. Granular deposits of IgA in dermal papillae.

Treatment

Dermatitis herpetiformis responds dramatically to sulphones. Dapsone is the drug of choice in most cases. Its use, however, is restricted by its side-effects, because it induces haemolysis, especially at higher doses. Alternatives are sulphapyridine and sulphamethoxypyridazine. Patients in whom a gluten-sensitivity has been demonstrated should also be started on a gluten-free diet, because there may be an increased risk of gut lymphoma (similar to coeliac disease). Indeed, some patients may respond to diet alone.

Linear IgA disease

Occasionally, patients with a pemphigoid- or dermatitis herpetiformis-like presentation are found to have a linear band of IgA at the basement membrane on immunofluorescence. This is now generally considered to be a

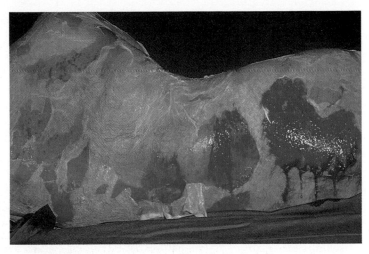

Fig. 14.12 Severe skin loss in toxic epidermal necrolysis.

separate bullous disease, which may be seen in both children and adults.

Rarer blistering diseases

Porphyria cutanea tarda

This is rare. It presents as small blisters and erosions on the backs of the hands, and on the forearms and face, following sun exposure or minor trauma. In many patients there is an underlying liver disorder, and often alcohol abuse.

Toxic epidermal necrolysis

This is a term applied to an acute disorder in which there is loss of the epidermis, usually over wide areas of the body surface (Fig. 14.12), although localized forms have been described. Nikolsky's sign is positive. Primary toxic epidermal necrolysis is usually an adverse reaction to a drug.

Extensive epidermal loss leads to severe dehydration and protein depletion. Patients require intensive care, and are best managed in a manner similar to those suffering from burns.

Bullous erythema multiforme (Stevens–Johnson syndrome)

This is a reactional state which may follow a wide variety of triggers (see Chapter 15). In severe erythema multiforme bullae may be the most prominent clinical feature.

CHAPTER 15

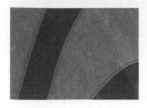

Miscellaneous Erythematous and Papulosquamous Disorders and Light-induced Skin Diseases

Miscellaneous: of mixed composition or character; of various kinds; many-sided. (Concise Oxford English Dictionary)

INTRODUCTION

This chapter is a mixed bag: it covers a number of common and/or important skin disorders which have not found a place elsewhere.

URTICARIA AND ANGIOEDEMA

Urticaria is the clinical term for a group of disorders characterized by the formation of 'weals'—swellings of the skin which disappear leaving no visible sign. Most of us have experienced one common form after falling (or being pushed) into nettles ('nettle-rash' is used commonly for urticaria). The basic pathology is dermal oedema due to vascular dilatation, often in response to histamine (and probably other mediators) released from mast cells.

Clinical features: the skin itches or stings; weals develop, white at first, then pink with a white rim; lesions can become very extensive and appear in many sites at once, but *always* clear spontaneously within a few hours, even though new lesions may continue to develop.

Typical lesions of urticaria are shown in Fig. 15.1.

A frequent accompanying feature of urticaria is *angioedema*, in which oedema extends into subcutaneous tissues. Sites of predilection are around the eyes, the lips, and in the oropharynx, which may swell alarmingly, occasionally resulting in complete closure of the eyes and compromising the airway.

Urticaria and angioedema may be part of a systemic anaphylactic reaction.

Clinical forms of urticaria and angioedema

Acute urticaria

Attacks last only a few hours or days. Common causes include:

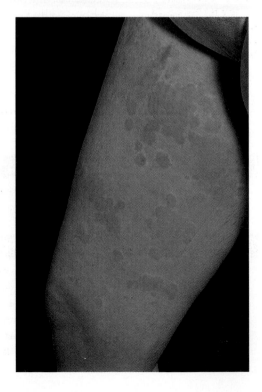

Fig. 15.1 Urticaria.

1 contact with plants (e.g. nettles), animal fur (dogs, cats, horses) or foods (milk, egg-white);

2 ingestion of foods, especially nuts, shellfish and strawberries;

3 ingestion of drugs, e.g. aspirin and penicillin.

Atopics are more susceptible. The reaction is generally triggered by immunoglobulin E (IgE) antibodies; some reactions, e.g. to aspirin, are due to direct mast cell degranulation.

Chronic urticaria

Attacks last for weeks, months or years. Contrary to popular expectations, a single aetiological factor is seldom found in this form of urticaria. Chronic ingestion of food colourings and preservatives may be important, but in our experience (and that of others in the UK) this is only true of a minority of patients.

The physical urticarias

Several physical insults may trigger urticarial responses:

1 dermographism, in which weals appear after scratch-marks (Fig. 15.2); this may occur in isolation or with other forms of urticaria;

2 pressure (delayed), in which weals develop up to 24 hours after pressure is applied;

3 cholinergic urticaria affects young men, in whom sweating is accompanied by small white weals with a red halo on the upper trunk;

4 cold;

5 water;

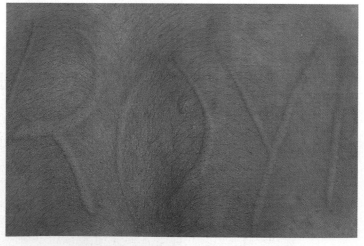

Fig. 15.2 Dermographism.

6 sunlight;

7 heat.

Hereditary angioedema

In this very rare autosomal dominant condition:

1 CI esterase inhibitor is lacking or defective;

2 there are sudden attacks of angioedema;

3 the gut may be affected.

Urticaria pigmentosa

Abnormal accumulations of mast cells give rise to multiple pigmented macules which urticate on being rubbed (see also Chapter 12).

Urticaria in systemic disease

An urticarial eruption may be part of a systemic disorder, especially hepatitis B. The rash seen in the evenings in Still's disease is also urticarial (see Chapter 19).

TREATMENT OF URTICARIA

If a possible trigger can be elicited from the history, it should be avoided. Aspirin should be banned in anyone prone to urticaria.

Most types of urticaria respond to H_1 antihistamines although some rarer forms are very resistant. A large range of agents is available, many of which cause CNS depression, but several newer antihistamines have little or no sedative effect (e.g. terfenadine, astemizole, loratidine). These are now drugs of first choice. It may help to add an H_2 antagonist (cimetidine, ranitidine).

It is sometimes necessary to use other agents, such as systemic steroids and adrenaline (see below).

TREATMENTS

- Acute attacks—a few days' treatment is usually sufficient
- Chronic urticaria—give a dose of antihistamine which suppresses the eruption completely; maintain this dose for several months; gradually withdraw treatment
- Angioedema—may require parenteral therapy with antihistamines, occasionally steroids
- Anaphylaxis—adrenaline and systemic steroids may be required
- Hereditary angioedema—does not respond to antihistamines or steroids; danazol works by increasing levels of the missing enzyme

ERYTHEMA MULTIFORME

The classic lesion of erythema multiforme is the 'iris' or 'target' lesion (Fig. 15.3), which is a round or oval area of erythema, with a dusky, purplish centre. Sometimes the centre becomes paler and a blister forms.

History: lesions appear suddenly, enlarge over the course of a few days, and then fade (often leaving pigmentary disturbances). The whole process settles in about 3 weeks. Repeated episodes are rare, but can be triggered by herpes simplex (see below).

Examination: the distribution characteristically includes extensor surfaces of arms and legs, but most important diagnostically is involvement of palms and soles.

Pathology: the process is a vasculitis and the more serious the vascular damage, the more dramatic are the changes. When really severe, the epidermis becomes necrotic and bullae may form.

Aetiology: erythema multiforme may occur out of the blue, but there are several recognized triggers.

TRIGGERS

- Herpes simplex—the commonest trigger; as herpes may be recurrent, so may herpes-related erythema multiforme
- Other viruses—orf, hepatitis, mumps
- Radiotherapy
- Cancers
- Connective tissue diseases
- A wide variety of drugs

Treatment: erythema multiforme is self-limiting, and treatment is not usually required.

Stevens–Johnson syndrome

At its most extreme erythema multiforme causes a major systemic disturbance. There is an acute onset, with severe inflammation of the conjunctivae, mouth and genitalia (Fig. 15.4), which may prevent normal eating, affect micturition, and cause ocular scarring. Patients occasionally die of severe bronchopulmonary involvement or renal failure.

Treatment: close attention must be given to fluid balance and nutrition. The role of systemic steroids is controversial, because the morbidity from steroids may outweigh that of the disease.

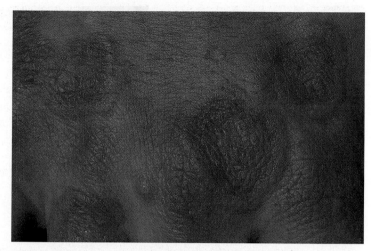

Fig. 15.3 'Target' lesion of erythema multiforme.

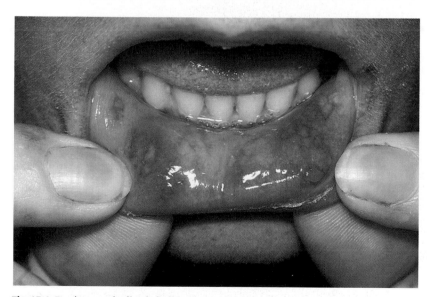

Fig. 15.4 Erosions on the lips in bullous erythema multiforme.

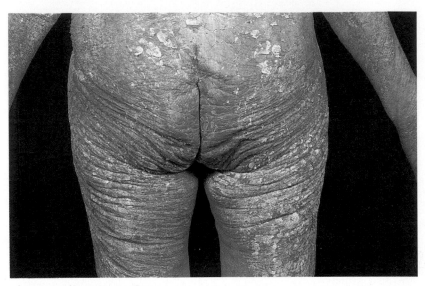

Fig. 15.5 Exfoliative dermatitis.

EXFOLIATIVE DERMATITIS (ERYTHRODERMA)

These terms (either will do) are used to describe a state in which most of the skin becomes red, inflamed and scaly (Fig. 15.5).

The four important causes of exfoliative dermatitis are as follows:

CAUSES

- Psoriasis
- Eczema/dermatitis
- Drug reactions
- Lymphomas (especially cutaneous T cell lymphoma)

The correct management depends on distinguishing between these causes, because the optimum treatment is different.

Clinical features: the skin is red, hot and scaly. There may be generalized lymphadenopathy. There is a loss of control of heat output, and there are bouts of shivering.

Effects: cardiac output is increased; protein is lost from the skin (and the gut); water loss from the skin is increased. Patients radiate heat into their surroundings, and there is a rise in metabolic rate, with mobilization of energy sources and increased muscle activity. The body cannot compensate for long, especially in the elderly.

Complications: cardiac failure; renal failure; sudden death due to central hypothermia.

Treatment.

1 Stop any potential causative drugs (see Chapter 21).

2 Nurse the patient in a warm room.

3 Attend to secondary medical problems (e.g. dehydration, heart failure and infections).

4 Biopsy skin to obtain definitive diagnosis.

5 Give short course of systemic steroids. If the diagnosis is known to be psoriasis from the outset, steroids should be avoided, and systemic antipsoriatic drugs used instead (see Chapter 8).

6 Initiate appropriate treatment for underlying diagnosis.

LICHEN PLANUS

Lichen planus is a rather variable disorder which probably affects 1% of new referrals to a dermatologist. The commonest pattern is an acute eruption of itchy papules (Fig. 15.6).

Sites of predilection: wrists, ankles and the small of the back; lichen planus may affect the mouth and genitalia.

Clinical features.

1 Skin lesions:
   (a) flat-topped;
   (b) shiny;
   (c) polygonal (Fig. 15.6).

2 Surface—fine network of dots or lines called 'Wickham's striae'.

3 Colour—'violaceous' (reddish-purple).

4 Oral—lacy, reticulate streaks on the cheeks (Fig. 15.7), gums and lips.

In the majority of patients, the eruption settles over a period of a few months. There are a number of variants, some of which are more persistent.

VARIANTS OF LICHEN PLANUS

- Hypertrophic: lichenified lumps appear on the legs
- Atrophic: largely seen in the mouth, lesions may be very chronic; small risk of carcinoma
- Follicular: may result in permanent scarring and hair loss
- Nail disease: nail changes may be very slight, or may lead to complete nail loss
- Drug-induced: see Chapter 21

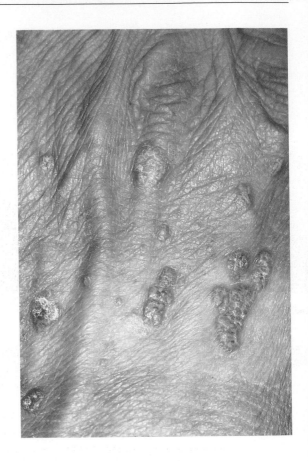

Fig. 15.6 Typical papules of lichen planus.

Aetiology: lichen planus appears to be a T cell-mediated attack on the epidermis. Similar changes are seen in graft-versus-host reactions. However, the cause of lichen planus in most instances remains a complete mystery.

Treatment: topical steroids usually suppress irritation; very extensive disease may need systemic steroids.

LICHEN NITIDUS

Probably a variant of lichen planus, this uncommon disorder produces clusters of tiny, asymptomatic papules.

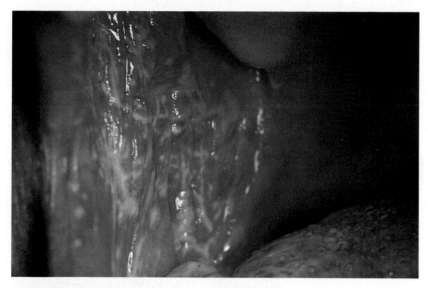

Fig. 15.7 Oral lesions in lichen planus.

LICHEN SCLEROSUS ET ATROPHICUS

Lichen sclerosus et atrophicus (often shortened to lichen sclerosus) is a disorder of unknown aetiology.

Note on terminology: there has been confusion in the terminology of vulval disease — gynaecologists and dermatologists have traditionally used different labelling systems. However, most authorities accept that lichen sclerosus has a special place in the nomenclature and is considered a specific entity.

Sites of predilection: the genitalia, especially in women.

Clinical features:

1 white, atrophic patches on the vulva, perineum and perianal skin;

2 similar plaques may develop elsewhere;

3 purpura and blistering may appear;

4 vulval lichen sclerosus easily becomes eroded and haemorrhagic, with severe soreness and irritation.

Complications: vulvo-vaginal stenosis; neoplastic change.

Childhood disease: lichen sclerosus in prepubertal girls often presents with dysuria and pain on defecation. It has been misdiagnosed as sexual abuse, but lesions are usually easy to diagnose (Fig. 15.8), and parents and child can be reassured. the prognosis of childhood disease is good, as many probably clear at puberty.

Disease in males: lichen sclerosus may be seen on the glans and prepuce (sometimes called 'balanitis xerotica obliterans'), and can give rise to phimosis and meatal stenosis. A significant number of boys undergo circumcision because of phimosis due to lichen sclerosus. Extra-genital lesions may also occur.

Treatment: the disease in adults generally pursues a chronic, relapsing course. Very potent topical steroids may provide symptomatic relief in vulval disease.

PITYRIASIS ROSEA

Pityriasis rosea is a self-limiting disorder, predominantly affecting children and young adults.

Clinical features.

I There may be a mild prodromal illness.

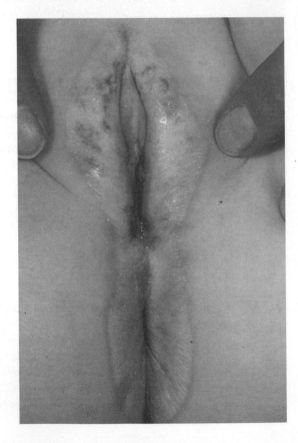

Fig. 15.8 Lichen sclerosus in a prepubertal girl.

2 One or more 'herald patches' appear. A herald patch is large, red, oval and scaly, and usually appears on the trunk or upper arm (it is often mis-diagnosed, especially as ringworm!).

3 A few days later, there is a sudden eruption of pink, oval patches on the trunk, upper arms and thighs.

There are three especially notable features.

1 On the trunk, lesions tend to lie with their long axes in lines sweeping from the back to the front (almost as if they were following spinal nerves).

This is said to look like an 'inverted Christmas tree' (Fig. 15.9) — but that depends on whether you are looking at the patient's back or front and on your concept of a Christmas tree! However, once understood, this sign will never be forgotten and *no other disorder produces this.*

2 The scale on the surface of each lesion exhibits a tendency to peel from the inside towards the edge, resulting in a so-called 'peripheral collarette' (Fig. 15.10).

3 If none of this has resulted in the diagnosis being made, it becomes clear when the rash disappears (as it always does) in 6–8 weeks.

Treatment: usually unnecessary, but mild topical steroids may help to relieve irritation.

Atypical pityriasis rosea: there may be no gap between the herald patch and the generalized rash; the eruption may extend down the arms and

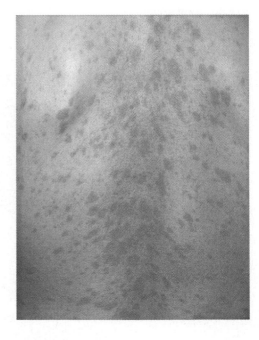

Fig. 15.9 Pityriasis rosea.

legs, and occasionally spares the trunk altogether; lesions may be so numerous that the distribution described above is not apparent; the inflammation may be so intense that it causes blisters.

PITYRIASIS LICHENOIDES

Small brownish-red papules surmounted by a 'plate' of scale appear on the trunk and limbs. Some patients have more acutely inflamed lesions which heal to leave pock marks.

PITYRIASIS RUBRA PILARIS

Pityriasis rubra pilaris (PRP) occurs in localized or generalized forms. All types are rare. Lesions are reddish-orange, and hair follicles are prominently involved. Generalized change is a very rare cause of exfoliative dermatitis (see above).

MILIARIA OR 'PRICKLY HEAT'

This is the exotic name for little red bumps which some people develop in hot humid conditions. It is due to sweat duct obstruction. It should not be confused with polymorphic light eruption (see below) in which the lesions are induced by light *not* heat. The condition is also seen in infants, particularly in the napkin area.

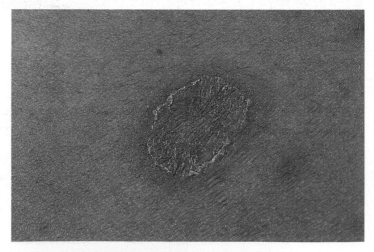

Fig. 15.10 Pityriasis rosea: the 'peripheral collarette' of scale.

PREGNANCY RASHES

Pregnancy may alter the course of a number of skin disorders, such as acne, eczema, psoriasis and vulval warts, and it may trigger erythema multiforme.

There are also three important conditions related to pregnancy itself.

CONDITIONS

Pruritus of pregnancy
• Up to 20% of women; may be due to oestrogen-induced cholestasis

Polymorphic eruption of pregnancy
• Blotchy, urticarial and papular rash with intense itching
• Onset in third trimester
• Lesions favour abdomen
• Particular predilection for striae (Fig. 15.11)
• Fades shortly after delivery

Herpes (pemphigoid) gestationis
• Blisters on urticated background
• Variant of bullous pemphigoid
• Rare

LIGHT-INDUCED SKIN DISEASE

But yet the light that led astray
Was light from Heaven
(Robert Burns, *The Vision*)

Sunlight is often thought to be beneficial: adverts for sunbeds, solaria and foreign holidays all bear witness to this twentieth century myth. However, ultraviolet radiation (UVR) can initiate, wholly or in part, many unwanted skin changes.

Some are chronic: cancers and keratoses (see Chapter 9); the yellowing, coarsening and wrinkling known as 'photo-ageing'. Note that most of today's tanned beauties are tomorrow's wrinkled prunes!

Some are more acute: sunburn; reactions to a combination of plants or drugs and light.

Some are due to metabolic disturbances, whereas in others the cause is quite unknown.

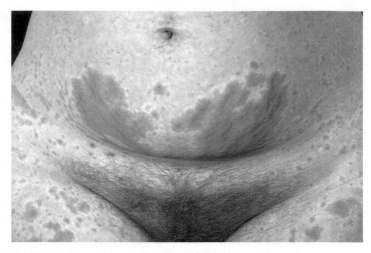

Fig. 15.11 Polymorphic eruption of pregnancy.

UVR may also exacerbate certain pre-existing skin disorders (see 'unwanted cutaneous reactions to light' below).

Sunburn

Most of us are familiar with sunburn, even if we have only seen it in others. Excessive medium wavelength UVR induces erythema and, if severe, blistering. The dose required depends on skin type (see Chapter 12), and the

UNWANTED CUTANEOUS REACTIONS TO LIGHT

- Sunburn
- Polymorphic light eruption
- Solar urticaria (see above)
- Actinic prurigo
- Juvenile spring eruption
- Hydroa vacciniforme
- Photosensitive eczema
- Porphyrias
- Pellagra
- Xeroderma pigmentosum
- Phytophotodermatitis
- Drug reactions

intensity of the UVR: skin types I and II are very prone to sunburn; sunlight around midday is the most intense.

Treatment of established sunburn is difficult, but calamine lotion and topical steroids may help symptomatically. Prevention is much better than cure.

Sun care should include avoidance, hats and clothing, sunglasses and sunscreens. All exposed surfaces need to be covered. Sunscreens come in a range of potencies, graded by 'Sun Protection Factor' (SPF) number. This number indicates the approximate multiple of time to redness that the screen will provide. If that is 10 minutes, a screen with SPF 6 will prolong this to about an hour.

Polymorphic light eruption

This common disorder is frequently misdiagnosed as 'prickly heat' (see above). Women are affected more often than men, and typically trouble starts in adolescence or early adulthood.

Clinical features: an eruption develops on light-exposed surfaces, most commonly the face, arms, legs, and the 'V' of the neck. Individual lesions vary from papules to plaques. Blisters are sometimes seen. The reaction may only occur in very strong sunlight, but even mild British summer sunshine can be the trigger.

Treatment: preseason PUVA is helpful. Antimalarials may be of some benefit, and sunscreens and clothing will help prevent the eruption in some.

Actinic prurigo

Actinic prurigo is a rare disorder of childhood in which eczematous areas develop on the face and backs of the hands every summer, and disappear in the winter. The cause is unknown and attempted treatment is often ineffective.

Juvenile spring eruption

Little boys occasionally develop blisters on the ears in the spring, and this is given the grand title of 'juvenile spring eruption'. It is probably a variant of polymorphic light eruption.

Photosensitive eczema and chronic actinic dermatitis

Some individuals develop eczema of light-exposed surfaces which clears in the winter months. In others a pre-existing eczema becomes much worse on exposure to light.

One cause is a contact dermatitis to airborne chemicals, such as perfumes or plant extracts (e.g. chrysanthemums). A similar picture may occur with certain drugs.

The changes tend to become more intense until the skin is permanently thickened and inflamed. This state is termed 'chronic actinic dermatitis'.

Treatment: this is very difficult. Barrier sunscreens containing titanium may help, and azathioprine has been shown to be of benefit.

Porphyrias

This miscellaneous group of disorders are due to enzyme defects in the haem production pathways. Some, but not all, are associated with photosensitivity.

The commonest in northern Europe is erythropoietic protoporphyria, in which burning in the sun (even through glass) develops in early childhood.

A form known as 'variegate porphyria' is seen in some Dutch and South African families.

It is perhaps worth mentioning that one of the rarest (congenital erythropoietic porphyria or Gunther's disease) may be the origin of the werewolf legend. Sufferers become disfigured and hairy, and they are anaemic (hence the werewolf's craving for blood). They avoid sunlight because of severe photosensitivity (the werewolf prowls at night when the moon is full—a logical time to prowl if there is no other source of illumination).

Pellagra

A photosensitive rash in the malnourished should suggest pellagra. The classical triad of diarrhoea, dermatitis and dementia is only seen in western societies in alcoholics and recluses.

Xeroderma pigmentosum

This rare disorder often presents with photosensitivity in early childhood (see also Chapter 11).

Phytophotodermatitis

Every summer, we see patients who have developed a rash following contact with plants on sunny days. Linear, streaky dermatitis (Fig. 15.12) results, and residual pigmentary disturbances are common. One important cause is giant hogweed, but there are several others.

Light-induced drug reactions

Several groups of drugs are associated with photoallergic and phototoxic reactions (see Chapter 21).

Disorders exacerbated by light

There are also a number of disorders which may show a deterioration or provocation on exposure to light (see 'disorders' on p. 218).

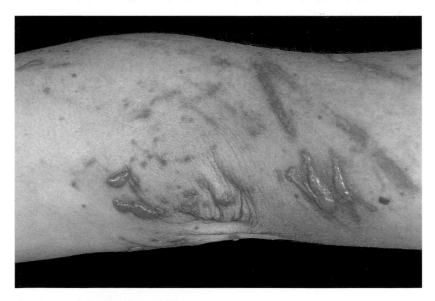

Fig. 15.12 A phytophotodermatitis.

DISORDERS

- Lupus erythematosus
- Rosacea
- Psoriasis
- Darier's disease
- Herpes simplex

The mechanisms for this are unclear.

CHAPTER 16

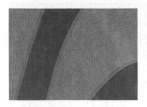

Vascular Disorders

LEG ULCERS

By far the commonest type of leg ulcer is the venous ulcer. Other causes of leg ulceration include ischaemia, vasculitis, skin neoplasia, and certain haematological disorders.

Venous hypertension and venous leg ulcers (varicose ulcers; gravitational ulcers)

Venous return from the legs is dependent on the calf muscles. When these muscles contract they pump blood in the deep veins towards the heart against gravity. Valves in the deep veins prevent reflux of blood when the calf muscles relax. During relaxation of the calf muscles blood passes from the superficial veins into the deep veins via perforating veins. If the valves in the deep and perforating veins are incompetent the calf muscle pump cannot function effectively and venous hypertension develops. Congenital abnormalities of the venous system, and valve damage following deep vein thrombosis, may contribute to incompetence. Genetic factors are probably also important.

The high pressure in the deep veins of the legs is transmitted via incompetent perforating veins to the superficial venous system (resulting in 'varicose' veins), and eventually to the capillary network. Skin capillaries become dilated, tortuous, and 'leaky'. Plasma passes through the vascular endothelium into the tissues, where fibrin forms cuffs around blood vessels. It is also possible that leucocyte stasis in capillaries leads to release of enzymes which damage vascular endothelium, increasing its permeability, and that this mechanism contributes to vessel leakage. These abnormalities impair the transfer of oxygen and nutrients, and the relatively devitalized tissue is susceptible to ulceration, either spontaneously or following minor trauma.

Problems caused by venous hypertension usually present in middle or old age, and women, particularly the obese, are predominantly affected. The clinical features are as follows.

VENOUS HYPERTENSION: CLINICAL FEATURES

- Varicose veins
- Oedema
- Lipodermatosclerosis
- Hyperpigmentation
- Eczema
- Atrophie blanche
- Ulceration

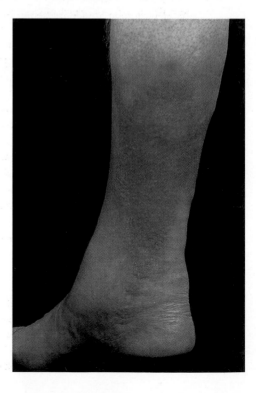

Fig. 16.1 Lipodermatosclerosis.

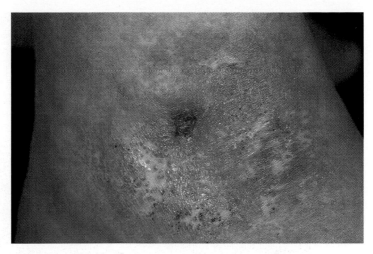

Fig. 16.2 Atrophie blanche.

Lipodermatosclerosis. This term refers to areas of induration, caused by fibrosis, on the lower parts of the legs, above the ankles (Fig. 16.1). There is initially an area of erythema, and this subsequently becomes purple–brown in colour. The tissues above the ankle are constricted, giving the leg the classical 'inverted champagne bottle' appearance.

Hyperpigmentation. Haemosiderin, derived from extravasated red cells, produces brown discolouration.

Eczema. Areas of 'varicose' eczema are common.

Atrophie blanche. This term is applied to areas of scar tissue within which are prominent dilated capillaries. Scattered pink dots are seen on a white background (Fig. 16.2). Such areas are very prone to ulcerate, and the ulcers are usually extremely painful.

Ulcers. The commonest site for a venous ulcer is the medial aspect of the leg, just above the medial malleolus, but the lateral malleolar area may also be affected (Fig. 16.3).

Rarely, a squamous cell epithelioma may develop in a long-standing venous ulcer.

TREATMENT

Lipodermatosclerosis may respond to early use of fibrinolysis-enhancing agents. Varicose eczema may be treated with mild potency topical steroids or medicated bandages containing zinc paste, zinc paste, calamine and clioquinol, or zinc paste and ichthammol. Potassium permanganate soaks are useful in the management of severe exudative eczema.

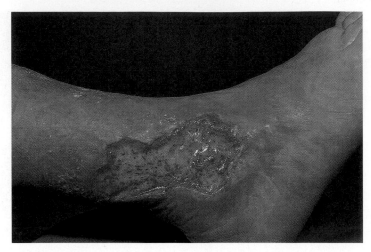

Fig. 16.3 Venous ulcer.

The most important aspect of ulcer management is to reduce venous hypertension and oedema by compression bandaging. Too much attention is paid to topical therapy of the ulcer, and not enough to increasing the efficiency of the calf muscle pump and eliminating oedema. This is just as vital after the ulcers have healed, but is often neglected, with the result that ulcers rapidly recur. However, it is essential to establish that the arterial blood supply to a limb is adequate (by Doppler studies) before using compression bandaging.

Secondary infection, often with a mixed bacterial flora, occurs in the majority of venous ulcers. However, systemic antibiotic therapy is not necessary unless there is associated cellulitis.

Adherent slough may be removed with tweezers and scissors, or by using a desloughing agent such as streptokinase/streptodornase solution.

There are numerous agents which have been marketed as topical therapies for leg ulcers. However, a simple regimen of regular cleansing with saline, followed by application of a topical antibacterial dressing such as chlorhexidine gauze, is usually adequate if combined with compression bandaging.

When an ulcer is clean and granulating, healing may be accelerated by grafting. A simple type of skin grafting procedure is pinch-grafting, in which small pieces of skin, usually taken from the thigh, are scattered over the surface of the ulcer (Fig. 16.4). The end result is a rather mammillated surface, but the cosmetic appearance is not important. Larger ulcers require more extensive partial-thickness grafting.

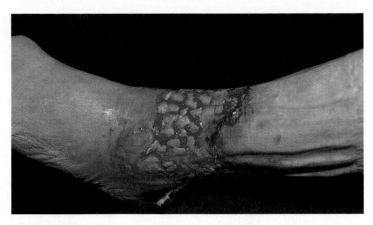

Fig. 16.4 Pinch grafts on a venous ulcer.

Weight reduction in the obese should also help, but this is extremely difficult to achieve. Vein surgery is only of value in a small number of cases.

Ischaemic ulcers

Ischaemic ulceration is usually a manifestation of atherosclerotic peripheral vascular disease. Typically, ischaemic ulcers occur on the dorsum or the sides of the foot, between the toes, or on the heel. Pedal pulses are reduced or absent, and Doppler studies will demonstrate impaired blood flow. Ischaemic ulcers are usually painful.

TREATMENT

The advice of a vascular surgeon should always be sought. In some cases the abnormalities can be treated and the viability of a limb preserved.

Vasculitic ulcers

Necrotizing vasculitis associated with a number of disorders, including rheumatoid arthritis and systemic lupus erythematosus (SLE), may produce leg ulcers.

Neoplastic ulcers

Basal cell carcinomas and squamous cell carcinomas arising on the legs may be mistaken for venous leg ulcers. However, they usually occur above the ankle region. If there is any doubt, a biopsy should be performed.

Haematological disorders and leg ulcers

Uncommon causes of leg ulcers include hereditary spherocytosis, sickle cell anaemia and thalassaemia. The mechanism of ulceration in these conditions is related to tissue hypoxia due to blockage of skin capillaries by abnormally shaped red cells.

VASCULITIS

Vascular inflammation may be classified according to the type of immunological reaction responsible for its production, the clinical appearance of the lesions, or the pathological changes visible on histology. As a result, it is easy to become completely confused by terminology.

Immunologically, type III (immune complex) and type IV (cell-mediated; delayed hypersensitivity) reactions are responsible for the majority of vasculitic disease. Clinically, vasculitis may present as urticaria, livedo reticularis, purpuric papules, nodules, haemorrhagic bullae or ulcers. Histologically, the changes are related to the immunological mechanisms responsible for the reaction, and can be classified as leucocytoclastic (immune complex-mediated; polymorphs predominate in the infiltrate), lymphocytic (delayed hypersensitivity; lymphocytes predominate), and granulomatous (immune complex-mediated; perivascular granuloma formation).

Clinical presentations of vasculitis

'ALLERGIC' VASCULITIS (LEUCOCYTOCLASTIC VASCULITIS)

Typically, an affected individual presents with numerous palpable, purpuric lesions on the legs, predominantly below the knees (Fig. 16.5). Some lesions may develop into haemorrhagic vesicles or bullae.

Histologically, there is fibrinoid necrosis of small blood vessels, and a perivascular infiltrate composed predominantly of neutrophil polymorphs. The perivascular tissues also contain extravasated red cells, and fragments of polymorph nuclei ('nuclear dust'). These changes are initiated by deposition of immune complexes in small vessels, complement activation, and production of polymorph chemotactic factors. Polymorphs attracted to the area release lysosomal enzymes which damage the vessel wall. Drugs, and bacterial or viral infections may act as the antigenic triggers for this type of reaction, but often the initiating factor is not discovered. This type of vasculitis may also be associated with rheumatoid arthritis, SLE and Sjögren's syndrome.

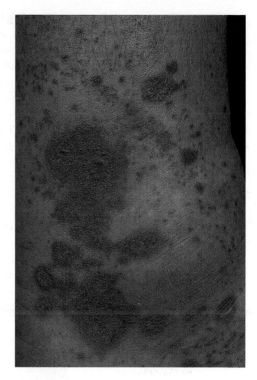

Fig. 16.5 Allergic vasculitis.

In many cases there is no evidence of systemic vascular involvement, but the joints, kidneys and gastrointestinal tract may be affected.

Henoch–Schönlein purpura (anaphylactoid purpura) is the name which has been given to a systemic allergic vasculitis occurring predominantly in children. Palpable purpuric lesions on the buttocks and legs are associated with arthralgia, vomiting and bloody diarrhoea, and proliferative glomerulonephritis. In many cases the precipitating factor appears to be a streptococcal sore throat.

Treatment

A period of bed rest may result in complete resolution of the skin lesions. In some cases, however, recurrent crops of lesions occur, and these may respond to therapy with dapsone. Dapsone does not affect immune complex formation, it simply blocks the pathomechanics of the production of skin lesions. In more severe cases, particularly those with systemic involvement, systemic steroid therapy may be necessary.

POLYARTERITIS NODOSA

Polyarteritis nodosa (also known as periarteritis nodosa) is an uncommon type of necrotizing vasculitis which affects medium-sized arteries throughout the body. Its aetiology is unknown in the majority of cases, but it may be provoked by hepatitis B infection. Middle-aged men are affected predominantly. Vessel damage results in aneurysm formation. Manifestations include pyrexia, weight loss, arthralgia and myalgia. Most affected individuals have a mild anaemia, leucocytosis, eosinophilia, and a high erythrocyte sedimentation rate (ESR) or raised plasma viscosity. Skin lesions include nodules (produced by vasculitis affecting small and medium-sized arteries), livedo reticularis, and ulcers.

There is a type of polyarteritis nodosa which affects the skin alone. Cutaneous nodules and livedo reticularis occur on the legs, usually below the knees, and there is no evidence of systemic involvement.

Treatment

Polyarteritis nodosa is treated with systemic steroids and immunosuppressive drugs.

ERYTHEMA NODOSUM

This condition usually affects children and young adults, and is characterized by the development of multiple tender, erythematous nodules, usually

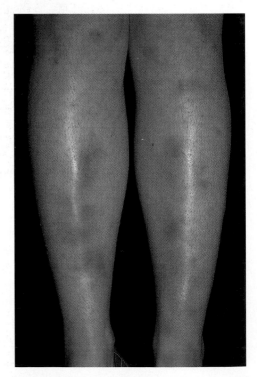

Fig. 16.6 Erythema nodosum.

on the shins (Fig. 16.6), but occasionally also on the forearms. As each nodule regresses it changes colour from red to purple to yellow–green— like a fading bruise. Pathologically, erythema nodosum is a nodular panniculitis associated with a lymphocytic vasculitis.

Causes of erythema nodosum include:

CAUSES

- Streptococcal infection
- Drugs: particularly sulphonamides , OCP also .
- Sarcoidosis
- Primary tuberculosis
- Inflammatory bowel disease

In some cases no precipitating factor is discovered

Investigation of a patient suffering from erythema nodosum should include culture of a throat swab, anti-streptolysin titre, chest X-ray, and Mantoux test.

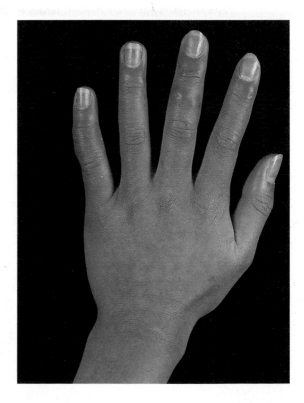

Fig. 16.7 Chilblains.

Treatment

In most cases bed rest and simple analgesia is all that is required. The lesions will gradually resolve over a period of a few days.

TEMPORAL ARTERITIS (GIANT CELL ARTERITIS)

Skin changes are rare, but ulceration may occur on the temporal and parietal regions of the scalp.

WEGENER'S GRANULOMATOSIS

This is a rare form of necrotizing granulomatous vasculitis affecting principally the small arteries of the respiratory tract, and associated with glomerulonephritis. Skin lesions take the form of a nodular vasculitis, sometimes with ulceration.

PYODERMA GANGRENOSUM

See Chapter 19.

BEHÇET'S SYNDROME

The principal features of this disorder are recurrent oral and genital ulceration and uveitis. Skin lesions include erythema nodosum and pustules at sites of minor trauma such as venepuncture sites.

PERNIOSIS (CHILBLAINS)

Chilblains are painful, inflammatory lesions provoked by exposure to cold (Fig. 16.7). The commonest sites for chilblains are the fingers and toes, but they may also occur on fatty prominences such as the fat pads on the medial aspects of the knees, and on the thighs. A characteristic type of perniosis occurs during winter months on the lateral aspect of the thighs of horse riders (equestrian cold panniculitis).

Treatment for chilblains is not very satisfactory, the best management being prophylaxis, by wearing warm gloves and thick socks, and, in the case of the equestrian, thermal underwear.

CHAPTER 17

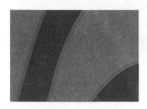

Connective Tissue Disorders

LUPUS ERYTHEMATOSUS

Lupus erythematosus is an autoimmune disorder which occurs in two main forms, systemic lupus erythematosus (SLE) which affects both the skin and internal organs, and discoid lupus erythematosus (DLE) in which the skin alone is affected. A small proportion of patients suffering from DLE may subsequently develop SLE. A third variant, subacute cutaneous lupus erythematosus (SCLE), is characterized by distinctive skin lesions which may be associated with systemic features.

Systemic lupus erythematosus

This is a multisystem disorder which may affect the skin, joints, heart and pericardium, lungs, kidneys, brain and haemopoietic system. Typically, the disease affects women, particularly of childbearing age, and progresses in a series of exacerbations and remissions. Its aetiology is unknown.

Mucocutaneous lesions include oropharyngeal ulceration, diffuse alopecia, Raynaud's phenomenon, and photosensitivity. Often there is facial erythema in a 'butterfly' distribution (Fig. 17.1). The 'butterfly' is represented by erythema on the cheeks linked by a band of erythema across the nose. However, by far the commonest cause of butterfly erythema is rosacea. Cutaneous vasculitis occurs in SLE, and microinfarcts on the digits, vasculitic lesions on the legs, or an urticaria-like eruption may occur.

Systemic manifestations include the following:

MANIFESTATIONS OF SLE

Polyserositis
- Arthralgia and arthritis (usually non-erosive)
- Pericarditis
- Pleurisy with effusions

Glomerulonephritis

Central nervous system involvement
- Psychosis and convulsions

Haemopoietic abnormalities
- Normochromic, normocytic anaemia
- Coombs' positive haemolytic anaemia
- Leucopenia
- Thrombocytopenia (associated with antiplatelet antibodies)

Pyrexia, weight loss and general malaise

INVESTIGATIONS

Anti-nuclear antibodies (ANA), also known as anti-nuclear factor (ANF), and DNA antibodies are found in most patients with SLE. Antibodies to double-stranded DNA are characteristic. A number of other autoantibodies may also occur in SLE, including anti-Ro, anti-La, antibodies to extractable nuclear antigen, lymphocytotoxic antibodies, and the lupus anticoagulant. A positive rheumatoid factor and biological false positive serological tests for syphilis may also be found.

Direct immunofluorescence study of clinically involved skin shows linear deposition of immunoglobulin G (IgG) or immunoglobulin M (IgM) and C3 at the dermoepidermal junction. Immunoglobulin and complement deposition may also be demonstrable in normal skin in light-exposed areas.

TREATMENT

Mild SLE may be managed with non-steroidal anti-inflammatory drugs or antimalarial therapy. Severe SLE will require treatment with systemic steroids and immunosuppressive agents. Plasmapheresis may also produce temporary benefit in severe cases. Light-exposed areas of skin should be protected by sunscreens with a high sun protection factor (SPF).

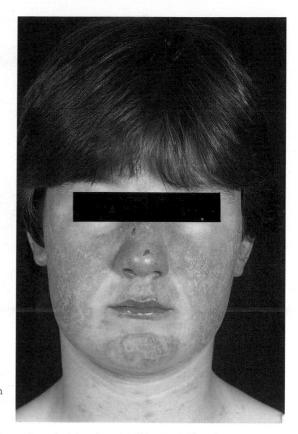

Fig. 17.1 Facial erythema in systemic lupus erythematosus.

PROGNOSIS

Severe renal and central nervous system involvement are poor prognostic factors, but for the majority of patients the prognosis is good.

DRUG-INDUCED SYSTEMIC LUPUS ERYTHEMATOSUS

Drug-induced SLE is rare. The drugs most frequently implicated in its provocation include hydralazine, procainamide, anticonvulsants (phenytoin, primidone), isoniazid and chlorpromazine.

Discoid lupus erythematosus

Classically, DLE affects light-exposed areas—principally the face and neck, but also the dorsa of the hands and the arms. Lesions may be precipitated or exacerbated by sunlight. Individual lesions consist of scaling, erythema-

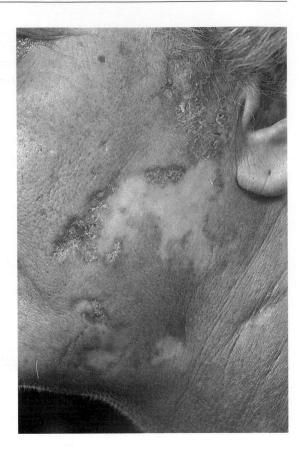

Fig. 17.2 Discoid lupus
erythematosus.

tous plaques, with prominent follicular plugging. If the scale is lifted off, follicular plugs may be seen on its undersurface — the so-called 'carpet-tack' sign. There may be only a few lesions, but extensive, cosmetically disfiguring involvement of the facial skin can occur. Lesions heal with scarring, and the typical picture is of an active, erythematous scaly margin enclosing a central area of scarred, hypopigmented, atrophic skin (Fig. 17.2). The scalp may be involved, producing areas of scarring alopecia in which follicles are permanently destroyed. Occasionally the buccal or nasal mucosae are affected.

INVESTIGATIONS

The diagnosis can be confirmed by skin biopsy. Histology shows a periadnexal lymphocytic infiltrate, liquefaction degeneration of the basal layer of

the epidermis, follicular plugging, and hyperkeratosis. Direct immunofluorescence of lesional skin reveals the same pattern of immunoglobulin deposition seen in SLE (see above). The ANF may be positive, but DNA
antibodies are not present in significant amounts.

TREATMENT

Potent fluorinated topical steroids are helpful in many cases, but if they
are ineffective, intralesional injection of triamcinolone, or oral therapy
with the antimalarial hydroxychloroquine may be required. Light-exposed
areas should be protected by a sunscreen with a high SPF. Where
there is extensive involvement of facial skin, the use of camouflage
creams can produce a considerable improvement in the cosmetic
appearance.

Subacute cutaneous lupus erythematosus

Non-scarring, papulosquamous or annular lesions occur predominantly
on light-exposed areas. Associated systemic features may occur, but are
usually mild.

DERMATOMYOSITIS

Heliotrope
A flower resembling the pale violet,
Which, with the Sun, though rooted-fast, doth move
And, being changed, yet changeth not her love.
(Ovid)

Dermatomyositis is an autoimmune inflammatory disease of skin and
muscle which may occur in childhood or in adult life. There are differences
in the manifestations of the disease in these two age groups. Vasculitis and
the late development of calcinosis are features of the childhood disease
which are not seen in adults. In some adults dermatomyositis is associated
with systemic malignancy, whereas there is no association with malignancy
in the childhood disease.

SKIN

The skin changes are as follows:

SKIN CHANGES

- Violaceous erythema of the face and V-area of the neck (Fig. 17.3). This is said to resemble the colour of the heliotrope flower, and is referred to as 'heliotrope erythema'
- Periorbital oedema
- Erythema on the dorsa of the hands, and linear erythema on the dorsa of the fingers (Fig. 17.4). Erythematous papules (Gottron's papules) over the knuckles
- Prominent, ragged cuticles and dilated capillaries in the proximal nail folds (Fig. 17.5)
- Erythema over knees and elbows
- In childhood, cutaneous vasculitis leads to ulceration of the skin, particularly in the axillae and groins

MUSCLES

In some cases there is little evidence of any muscle disease, whereas in others there is profound muscle weakness. Typically, there is proximal,

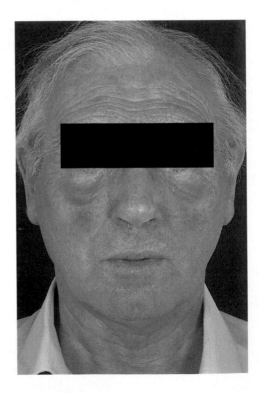

Fig. 17.3 Facial erythema in dermatomyositis.

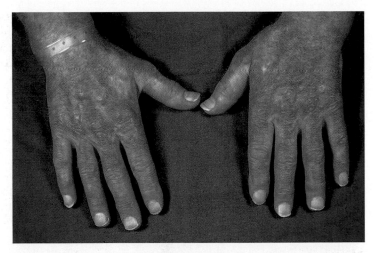

Fig. 17.4 Linear erythema on the dorsa of the hands in dermatomyositis.

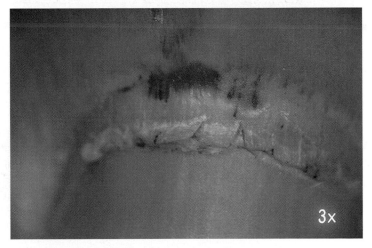

Fig. 17.5 Hypertrophic cuticle, and nail fold telangiectasia in dermatomyositis.

symmetrical weakness and wasting of the limb girdle muscles. Pharyngeal and oesophageal muscles may also be involved, leading to dysphagia.

Other features include pulmonary fibrosis, and arthralgia and/or arthritis.

There have been a number of studies of the association between adult dermatomyositis and systemic malignancy, and these have produced some controversy about the prevalence of this association. There is no doubt that some adult patients have an underlying systemic malignancy, but there is no general agreement as to how frequently this association occurs. Several studies have suggested that extensive screening for occult neoplasia is of little value. However, if a patient with dermatomyositis develops pulmonary or abdominal symptomatology this should be thoroughly investigated.

Investigations

Electromyography and biopsy of affected muscles, measurement of serum enzymes (creatine kinase; aldolase) derived from muscle, and a 24-hour urine creatine level will help to confirm the diagnosis.

Treatment

In dermatomyositis associated with malignancy, there is usually marked improvement when the neoplasm is excised. A relapse of the dermatomyositis signals a recurrence.

The mainstay of therapy is oral corticosteroids. If the response to steroids is poor, immunosuppressives such as azathioprine, methotrexate, cyclophosphamide or chlorambucil may be of benefit. Where there is severe muscle involvement, physiotherapy is an important adjunct to drug therapy, in order to minimize contractures.

SCLERODERMA

Scleroderma means 'thickening of the skin', and is a term applied to a group of diseases in which there is sclerosis of the skin and destruction of hair follicles and sweat glands. Scleroderma may be an isolated cutaneous phenomenon, when it is called 'morphoea', or a cutaneous component of a multisystem disorder.

CLASSIFICATION OF SCLERODERMA

- Morphoea. Sclerosis of the skin without systemic involvement
- Systemic sclerosis. Cutaneous sclerosis in association with a vasculopathy of small arteries producing multi-organ systemic disease
- Chemically induced scleroderma. Sclerosis of the skin as a manifestation of the toxic effects of certain chemicals
- Pseudoscleroderma. Sclerosis of the skin associated with a number of diseases other than morphoea or systemic sclerosis

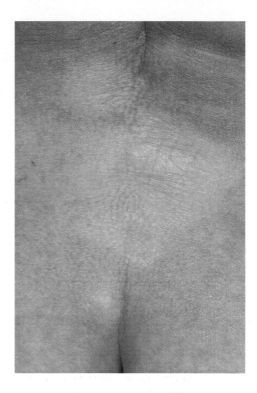

Fig. 17.6 A plaque of morphoea.

Morphoea

This is a disorder of unknown aetiology in which there is sclerosis of the skin. Morphoea may be subdivided clinically into the following types:

1 circumscribed;
2 linear;
3 frontoparietal (*en coup de sabre*);
4 generalized.

1 *Circumscribed.* This is the commonest clinical presentation of morphoea. Solitary or multiple indurated plaques develop, predominantly on the trunk. Initially, affected areas of skin have a violaceous hue, but gradually become thickened and ivory in colour (Fig. 17.6). The surface is smooth and shiny. Eventually, usually after many months, the sclerosis resolves, leaving atrophic, hyperpigmented areas.

2 *Linear.* Linear morphoea usually affects one limb, often extending its full length. In childhood, it can significantly impair the growth of the limb, and produce severe flexion deformities of large joints and digits.

3 *Frontoparietal (en coup de sabre).* Resembling a sabre cut across the scalp and forehead, this type of morphoea is a considerable cosmetic problem. A linear, depressed, sclerotic area extends from the face into the scalp, and is associated with loss of hair.

4 *Generalized.* There is extensive sclerosis of the skin of the trunk and limbs. Flexion contractures restrict limb movement, and if the chest is severely affected breathing may be impaired.

TREATMENT OF MORPHOEA

There is no effective treatment for morphoea. In linear morphoea on the limbs, physiotherapy is essential to maintain joint motility, and orthopaedic surgery may be necessary. Plastic surgery can be of benefit in frontoparietal morphoea.

The natural history of morphoea is gradual spontaneous resolution.

Systemic sclerosis

This is a condition of unknown aetiology in which sclerotic changes in the skin occur as one component of a multisystem disorder associated with a vasculopathy of small arteries. The skin changes affect predominantly the face and hands.

Persistent leg ulcers, predominantly affecting the ankles, are not uncommon in systemic sclerosis.

CUTANEOUS FEATURES OF SYSTEMIC SCLEROSIS

Face
- The facial skin is sclerotic and bound to underlying structures, producing a tight, shiny appearance, with loss of facial wrinkles, a beaked nose, and restriction of mouth opening (Fig. 17.7)
- Peri-oral furrowing ('purse-string mouth')
- Facial telangiectasia
- Loss of lip vermilion

Hands
- Raynaud's phenomenon
- Tight sclerotic skin producing progressive contractures of the digits (sclerodactyly)
- Finger pulp infarcts producing small, painful ulcers (Fig. 17.8). These infarctive changes lead to progressive pulp atrophy and resorption of the underlying terminal phalanges
- Calcinosis (Fig. 17.9)

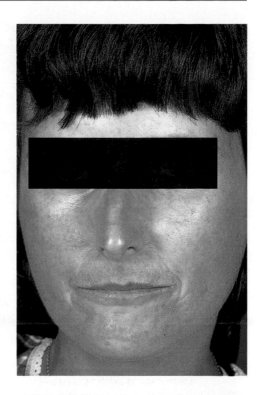

Fig. 17.7 Facial appearance in systemic sclerosis.

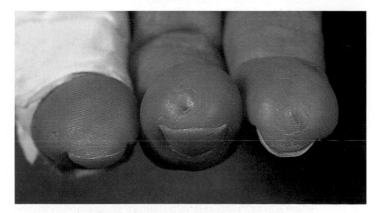

Fig. 17.8 Finger pulp ulcers and scars in systemic sclerosis.

SYSTEMIC INVOLVEMENT

Gastrointestinal. Atrophy and fibrosis of the circular smooth muscle of the oesophagus results in impaired peristalsis. The gastro-oesophageal sphincter mechanism is also impaired, leading to gastro-oesophageal reflux,

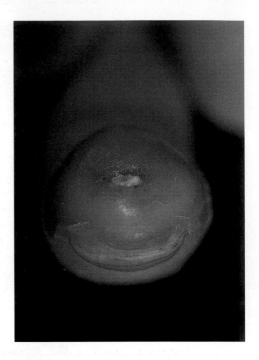

Fig. 17.9 Calcinosis in systemic sclerosis.

oesophagitis, and stricture formation. Symptoms of oesophageal reflux are common. Dysphagia usually indicates the development of oesophageal stricture. Barium swallow in the Trendelenberg position (head down) will demonstrate oesophageal dysfunction.

Atrophy and fibrosis of the smooth muscle of the small bowel leads to impaired peristalsis, and the resultant stagnation of small bowel contents predisposes to bacterial overgrowth. Gut bacteria deconjugate bile salts (which are essential for micelle formation) and this leads to fat malabsorption and steatorrhoea. Occasionally, patients present with a picture simulating acute intestinal obstruction.

The large bowel classically shows multiple wide-mouthed pseudodiverticula.

Pulmonary. Pulmonary disease develops insidiously, with increasing shortness of breath due to pulmonary fibrosis and pulmonary hypertension. The latter is due to disease of small pulmonary arteries, and eventually leads to cor pulmonale.

Renal. Fibrinoid changes in arteries and arterioles are associated with proteinuria and hypertension. Renal involvement is usually mild, but in a few cases it is rapidly progressive and leads to renal failure.

Nervous system. Neurological involvement is uncommon, but carpal tunnel syndrome and trigeminal neuropathy have been reported.

Cardiac. Myocardial fibrosis, conduction disorders and a variety of electrocardiographic (ECG) abnormalities have been described.

Hepatic. There is a significant association between systemic sclerosis and primary biliary cirrhosis.

Musculoskeletal. Arthralgia and arthritis occur in some patients, and myopathy and inflammatory myositis may also occur.

TREATMENT

Systemic steroid therapy is of no benefit in the majority of cases, unless there is an inflammatory myositis. Penicillamine is also usually ineffective. Digital ischaemia may be helped by electrically heated gloves and socks. Prostacyclins, ketanserin or nifedipine may help relieve Raynaud's phenomenon. Patients with symptoms of oesophageal reflux should avoid lying flat, and may benefit from antacids, H_2-receptor antagonists, and metoclopramide. A broad-spectrum antibiotic may help patients with malabsorption.

PROGNOSIS

Severe pulmonary or renal involvement are poor prognostic factors, but the majority of patients suffering from systemic sclerosis live for many years.

Chemically induced scleroderma

Polyvinyl chloride (PVC) can induce a disorder resembling idiopathic systemic sclerosis, and 'vinyl chloride disease' has been described in workers in the PVC industry, particularly reactor cleaners. A number of other chemicals may induce diseases mimicking systemic sclerosis, including perchlorethylene and trichlorethylene (solvents used in dry-cleaning), and bleomycin. A disorder similar to systemic sclerosis occurred in 1981 in people poisoned by contaminated rape-seed oil sold as cooking oil in Madrid.

Pseudoscleroderma

Scleroderma-like changes may be seen in a number of unrelated conditions, including porphyria cutanea tarda, carcinoid syndrome, and phenylketonuria.

CHAPTER 18

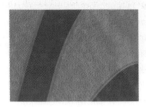

Pruritus

> *There was a young belle of old Natchez*
> *Whose garments were always in patches*
> *When comment arose*
> *On the state of her clothes*
> *She drawled: 'When ah itchez, ah scratchez!'*
> (Ogden Nash, *Requiem*)

Pruritus means itching. *Please* note the correct spelling: it is *not* spelt *pruritis* as often appears in student exam papers, clinical notes and referral letters!

Pruritus varies in its duration, localization, and severity. Everyone has experienced short-term, localized, itch, and there is a perverse joy in having a really good scratch. However, some individuals suffer from distressing chronic irritation lasting for years. Itching may be restricted to one or more sites, or cover virtually the whole body surface. It may creep about, appearing first on an arm and later on the back, or in more than one site simultaneously. Itching can be mild or appallingly severe, constant and distressing. Chronic pruritus can completely ruin the quality of life.

Pruritus is prominent in many skin diseases. Especially itchy are the eczemas, lichen planus, insect bites and infestations, urticaria and dermatitis herpetiformis. However, the skin may also itch when no cutaneous abnormality is visible.

MECHANISMS OF PRURITUS

We do not clearly understand why skin diseases itch, and we know very little about irritation in otherwise apparently normal skin.

An itch is produced, conditioned and appreciated at several levels in the nervous system: stimulus; mediators and receptors; peripheral pathways; central processing; interpretation. A wide variety of stimuli can induce an itch, and a number of chemicals may be involved in its production, especially histamine and some proteinases. Prostaglandins also enhance the itch sensation. However, the roles of these agents are obscure: although histamine can induce itch without wealing, non-sedative antihistamines have no effect on simple pruritus.

More complex, central mechanisms may also be important in modulating and appreciating pruritus. Many itch-provoking stimuli induce pain if applied at higher intensities. Indeed, scratching appears to induce pain and to abolish irritation. However, other sensory stimuli can also abolish itching, and more complex mechanisms have been proposed. One theory involves a complicated filtering system controlling input pathways to further stimuli and passing information on to higher centres.

Itching can certainly be affected by higher centres. It is much less apparent when the mind is fully occupied and much worse when boredom sets in. 'Stress' and other psychological factors can induce or worsen pruritus.

CAUSES OF PRURITUS

The term 'pruritus', used without qualification, implies that there is itching without a *primary* skin disorder. However, in many instances there are considerable *secondary* skin changes from scratching (e.g. excoriations, scars and prurigo—see below).

But watch out! Skin disorders with subtle changes can easily be obscured by scratching: a classical example of this is scabies (see Chapter 5). A full history and a careful examination of the skin are therefore important in all patients complaining of itching.

In considering causes, we shall look separately at localized itching, generalized states, and so-called 'senile' pruritus.

Localized pruritus

Localized irritation of the skin is common. The skin may be normal, but it is more common to find some abnormalities.

Two very important and troublesome forms of localized pruritus are lichen simplex chronicus and prurigo, and anogenital pruritus.

LICHEN SIMPLEX CHRONICUS AND PRURIGO

This difficult problem is sometimes labelled 'neurodermatitis'. Constant irritation leads to constant scratching which, in turn, leads to thickening of the skin. This may occur in plaques, known as lichen simplex chronicus (Fig. 18.1) or in nodules, which are given the name 'prurigo' (Fig. 18.2). The areas are irritable, and a self-perpetuating itch/scratch cycle develops. Patients who develop this kind of localized itching are often rather tense.

Sites of predilection: lichen simplex chronicus — classical sites include shins, forearms, palms and the back of the neck (sometimes known as 'lichen nuchae'); perianal and vulval skin may also be affected (see below). Prurigo nodules — may accompany areas of lichen simplex or appear separately almost anywhere; they are frequently multiple.

Lesions are often asymmetrical.

Treatment: potent topical steroids (sometimes under occlusive bandages) may help, but the problem often recurs.

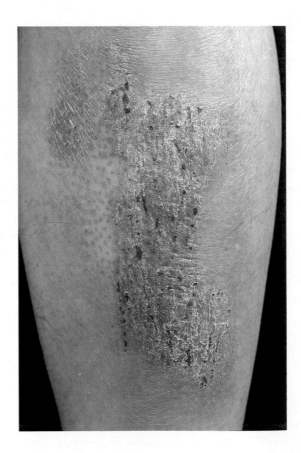

Fig. 18.1 Lichen simplex chronicus.

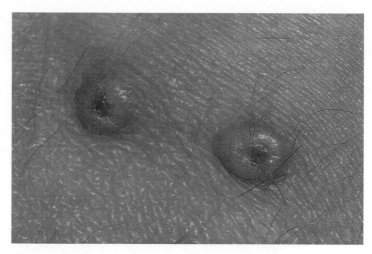

Fig. 18.2 Nodular prurigo.

ANOGENITAL PRURITUS

Two very common (and least talked about) forms of localized itching are pruritus vulvae and pruritus ani. They may be encountered together.

Pruritus ani is often attributed to haemorrhoids. However, although haemorrhoids and tags are often present, their treatment alone does not always relieve the symptoms. The problem is also often dismissed as psychological, but only rarely is this the complete explanation.

Anal itching may continue for years. Irritation is often spasmodic and extremely intense. The majority of patients are male.

Clinical features: examination often reveals little abnormality; there may be some excoriation and thickening of anal and perianal skin; 'tags' are often present; occasionally gross changes amounting to lichen simplex are seen; there may be an associated fissure.

Aetiology: pruritus ani is probably largely a low-grade irritant reaction to faeces, sweat and discharge; sedentary occupations make matters worse. Contact allergy to medicaments is common, especially to anaesthetics, preservatives and aminoglycosides. Psoriasis of the natal cleft and perineum may give rise to pruritus ani.

Pruritus vulvae can be very distressing. There are a number of causes to consider.

CAUSES

- Mild incontinence (with prolapse) may cause irritant changes
- Skin disorders: notably eczema, psoriasis and lichen sclerosus et atrophicus (see Chapter 15)
- Allergic contact dermatitis to medicaments (as in anal itch—see above)
- Candidosis (secondary to diabetes): the vulva is beefy red, and there may be pustules and a vaginal discharge
- Vulval itch with no visible signs, when a true 'psychogenic origin' is suspected

Treatment of perineal irritation depends upon the cause.

TREATMENT

'Irritant' pruritus ani
- Good hygiene, a high fibre diet, and treatment with topical steroids are useful
- Treating concomitant haemorrhoids may reduce discharge

Skin disorder and allergic contact dermatitis
- Most will require topical steroids (but see also relevant chapter)

Candidosis
- Antifungal creams and pessaries; check for diabetes

No changes seen
- Patients seldom respond to antipruritics
- Inexpert psychological probing is valueless

Generalized pruritus

Generalized pruritus is extremely unpleasant, and can either affect most of the body surface continuously or involve several different areas. By definition, a primary skin disorder has been excluded.

Clinical features: skin changes vary considerably—nothing to see at all; mild flakiness of the skin, with a few scratch marks; or the skin may be covered in excoriations, scars and nodules. The skin is often dry, especially in the elderly.

Although there may be no identifiable underlying disorder, all patients with generalized irritation should be investigated because a number of potentially remediable systemic disorders may be responsible.

SYSTEMIC DISORDERS

Haematological disorders
- Iron deficiency
- Polycythaemia rubra vera

Cholestatic liver disease
- Extrahepatic obstruction
- Primary biliary cirrhosis
- Hepatitis
- Drug-induced cholestasis

Chronic renal failure

Thyroid disease
- Thyrotoxicosis
- Myxoedema

Malignancy
- Lymphomas and leukaemias
- Carcinomas

Drug ingestion
- Especially opiates

Pregnancy (see Chapter 15)

HAEMATOLOGICAL DISORDERS

Chronic iron deficiency may be due to blood loss (e.g. from menorrhagia or a gut carcinoma). Many elderly patients and some vegans are iron deficient for dietary reasons. Polycythaemia rubra vera is characteristically associated with itching triggered by bathing.

LIVER DISEASE

The itch is probably related to bile salts in the skin. Irritation may precede the development of other features of cholestatic liver disease, especially in primary biliary cirrhosis.

CHRONIC RENAL FAILURE

Unfortunately the intractable itch is largely unaffected by dialysis. Parathyroidectomy may help, but the benefit is generally short-lived and is hardly justified in most patients.

THYROID DISEASE

Both thyrotoxicosis and myxoedema may present with pruritus. In myxoedema the general dryness of the skin may be responsible.

CANCERS

Lymphoreticular malignancies are particularly prone to cause itching, but pruritus may also occur in association with a variety of carcinomas. Up to 30% of Hodgkin's disease patients suffer from generalized pruritus.

DRUGS

Various agents induce itching, but the mechanisms are poorly understood. Opiates appear to act centrally and on mast cells. Oestrogens and phenothiazines induce cholestasis.

DIABETES MELLITUS

You may come across lists which quote diabetes as a cause of itching, but we do not consider that this is the case.

PSYCHOLOGICAL FACTORS

When everything else has been excluded, psychological factors may be considered. The most common underlying problem is an anxiety neurosis, but patients with monodelusional psychoses such as parasitophobia also itch. These individuals, however, offer their own explanation only too readily! (see Chapter 20).

Screening procedures for generalized pruritus are as follows:

SCREENING

- A full history and general examination
- Full blood count
- ESR (or plasma viscosity)
- Liver function tests
- Blood urea/urea nitrogen/creatinine
- Iron studies
- Serum thyroxine
- Urine protein
- Chest X-ray

If these tests are negative initially, and if the pruritus persists, repeat at intervals

- Also consider CT scanning to exclude lymphoma

TREATMENT

Treatment of generalized pruritus is that of its cause. When no apparent underlying reason can be found, a topical steroid and a sedative antihistamine, such as hydroxyzine, may help.

Senile pruritus and xerosis

Itching with no apparent cause is common in the elderly. It may be mild and localized, but can be very severe and generalized. The patients (and their carers) are often anxious and miserable, but this is usually secondary to the irritation rather than a primary cause. This state is called 'senile pruritus'. It is not known what causes ageing skin to itch.

EXAMINATION

The skin is texturally either 'normal' or 'dry'. Excoriations, secondary eczematization and areas of infection are common. Localized areas of 'eczema craquelé' may develop (see Chapter 7).

TREATMENT

Treatment is extremely difficult. Sedative antihistamines often cause excessive drowsiness and confusion, and topical steroids are of limited use.

If the skin is texturally 'dry', liberal use of emollients may be helpful. Care has to be taken, however, as these agents can make both the patient and their surroundings very slippery!

Increased frequency of washing or the use of harsh soaps and detergents makes matters worse, both by removing surface lipids and acting as direct irritants. Soaps should therefore be used sparingly and emollients employed instead.

CHAPTER 19

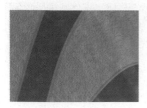

Systemic Disease and the Skin

The skin may be involved directly or indirectly in a number of systemic disease processes, and provide visible diagnostic clues leading to the discovery of internal disease.

ENDOCRINE DISEASE

Diabetes

There are a number of cutaneous manifestations of diabetes, including the following:

CUTANEOUS FEATURES

1 Certain cutaneous infections
2 Neuropathic ulcers
3 Necrobiosis lipoidica diabeticorum
4 Diabetic dermopathy
5 Bullosis diabeticorum
6 Xanthomata
7 Effects of insulin injections on the skin and subcutaneous tissues

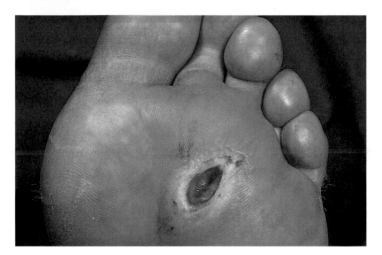

Fig. 19.1 Diabetic neuropathic ulcer.

I *Cutaneous infection.* Mucosal candidiasis, particularly balanitis and vulvo-vaginitis, tinea (pityriasis) versicolor, and carbuncles, occur more frequently in diabetics.

2 *Neuropathic ulcers.* Impaired sensation, as a result of sensory neuropathy, predisposes to the development of neuropathic ulcers on the soles of the feet (Fig. 19.1).

3 *Necrobiosis lipoidica diabeticorum.* Lesions of necrobiosis lipoidica characteristically occur on the shins, although they may develop elsewhere. The lesions are yellowish-brown and atrophic (Fig. 19.2).

Occasionally they ulcerate. Not all patients with necrobiosis lipoidica are diabetic (approximately 50% presenting with the skin lesions), and of the others, some will subsequently develop diabetes. Good diabetic control does not appear to influence the skin lesions.

Topical and intralesional steroids are used in the treatment of necrobiosis lipoidica, but results of treatment are not very impressive.

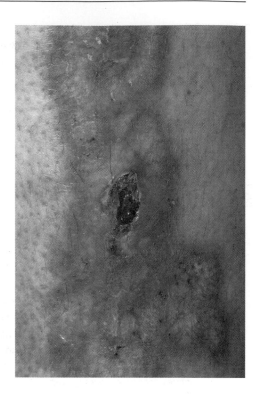

Fig. 19.2 Necrobiosis lipoidica
diabeticorum.

4 *Diabetic dermopathy.* This term is applied to small, brown, scar-like lesions seen on the shins in some diabetics. The lesions are thought to be associated with diabetic microangiopathy.

5 *Bullosis diabeticorum.* In this uncommon blistering disorder of diabetics subepidermal bullae occur on the hands and feet, without any obvious pre-existing inflammatory change. The aetiology of the blisters is unknown.

6 *Xanthomata.* Hyperlipidaemia in uncontrolled diabetes may be associated with the development of multiple small, yellow, eruptive xanthomata.

7 *Effects of insulin injections.* Insulin injections may cause lipoatrophy or fat hypertrophy ('insulin tumours') at injection sites.

MISCELLANEOUS

Other cutaneous manifestations include acanthosis nigricans in association with insulin-resistant diabetes; insulin-resistant diabetes associated with partial or generalized cutaneous lipoatrophy, and a scleroderma-like thickening of the skin of the hands (diabetic cheiroarthropathy) in insulin-dependent diabetics.

GRANULOMA ANNULARE

There is no significant association between classical granuloma annulare and diabetes, but in the much rarer generalized form of granuloma annulare there is a high incidence of diabetes. Typically, lesions of granuloma annulare are groups of firm, skin-coloured papules, often arranged in rings, and commonly occurring on the dorsa of the hands and feet (Fig. 19.3). The natural history of granuloma annulare is eventual spontaneous resolution, but persistent lesions may be treated with intralesional triamcinolone or cryotherapy.

THYROID DISEASE

Hypothyroidism

The skin is typically dry, and feels thickened due to subcutaneous mucin deposition—hence the designation myxoedema. A malar flush on an otherwise pale face produces what has been referred to as a 'strawberries and cream' appearance. There may be a yellowish tinge to the skin, said to be due to the deposition of carotenes. There is often peri-orbital oedema. The scalp hair is coarse and brittle, and there is loss of the outer part of the eyebrows. Sitting close to the fire to keep warm may produce severe erythema ab igne ('granny's tartan') on the shins.

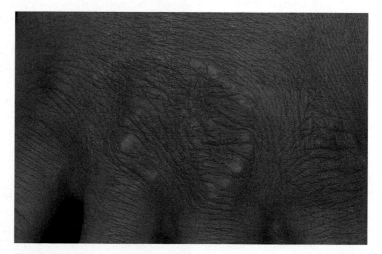

Fig. 19.3 Granuloma annulare.

Hyperthyroidism

Cutaneous changes which may accompany thyrotoxicosis include hyperhidrosis, palmar erythema, diffuse alopecia, generalized hyperpigmentation, and thyrotoxic acropachy (digital clubbing). The nails may show onycholysis. Some patients develop pretibial myxoedema, which is produced by subcutaneous deposition of excessive amounts of mucopolysaccharide, and is characterized by erythema and thickening of the soft tissues over the shins and dorsa of the feet (Fig. 19.4).

Vitiligo may accompany autoimmune thyroid disease, and generalized pruritus may be a feature of both hypothyroidism and hyperthyroidism.

ADRENAL DISEASE

Cushing's syndrome

The cutaneous effects of Cushing's syndrome include thinning of the skin,

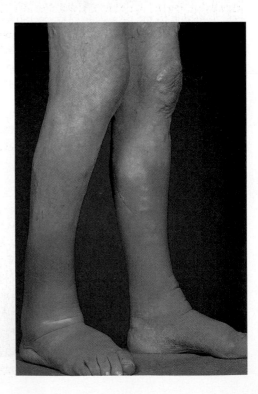

Fig. 19.4 Pretibial myxoedema.

spontaneous bruising, prominent purple striae on the trunk and limbs, diffuse alopecia, acne, and hirsutism.

Addison's disease

Diffuse hyperpigmentation is the main cutaneous manifestation of Addison's disease. The pigmentation is particularly prominent on the buccal mucosa and in the palmar creases. Vitiligo may also accompany autoimmune Addison's disease.

RHEUMATIC DISEASES

Gout

In addition to tophaceous deposits around affected joints, gouty tophi may occur on the ears.

Still's disease (systemic juvenile chronic arthritis)

This is a disorder of childhood, although it may rarely occur in adults. Accompanying the pyrexial episodes of Still's disease is a diffuse maculo-papular eruption which characteristically develops in the late afternoon and evening, and usually resolves by the following morning.

Rheumatoid arthritis

Dermatological features of rheumatoid arthritis include the following:

DERMATOLOGICAL FEATURES

- Rheumatoid nodules. Subcutaneous nodules over bony prominences, particularly on the extensor aspect of the forearms and the dorsa of the hands
- Vasculitic lesions. Digital vasculitis may produce small infarcts around the nail folds (Bywaters' lesions), or more severe digital ulceration and even gangrene. Vasculitic lesions may also occur on the legs, and contribute to the development of leg ulcers
- Pyoderma gangrenosum
- Palmar erythema

Rheumatic fever

Almost extinct in developed countries, rheumatic fever may be accompanied by a characteristic eruption, erythema marginatum.

Reiter's syndrome

Predominantly a disease of young adult males, Reiter's syndrome is usually precipitated by non-specific urethritis, but occasionally by bacillary dysentery. In addition to urethritis, conjunctivitis/uveitis, and arthritis, there may be an eruption which is indistinguishable from psoriasis. On the soles of the feet the skin lesions may become extremely thickened, producing so-called 'keratoderma blennorrhagicum' (see pp. 115–116). The buccal mucosa may show scattered erosions, and superficial circumferential erosive changes on the penis are referred to as 'circinate balanitis'.

VITAMIN DEFICIENCY

Scurvy

The classical picture of vitamin C (ascorbic acid) deficiency is rarely seen nowadays in developed countries, but scurvy may be encountered in the elderly and in alcoholics, as a result of nutritional self-neglect. The typical appearance is of perifollicular purpura, easy bruising, poor wound healing, bleeding gums, and woody oedema of the legs. The diagnosis can be confirmed by measuring leucocyte ascorbic acid levels.

Pellagra

Pellagra is the result of nicotinic acid deficiency. Classically, it has three major manifestations—dermatitis, diarrhoea and dementia. The dermatitis affects light-exposed areas, and there is often a well-demarcated margin to the affected area on the neck (Casal's necklace). Pellagra may occur in alcoholics as a result of nutritional self-neglect. A similar dermatitis may be provoked by isoniazid in individuals who are slow acetylators of this drug, and who also have a low dietary intake of vitamins.

INFLAMMATORY BOWEL DISEASE

Ulcerative colitis and Crohn's disease may be associated with a number of mucocutaneous manifestations including the following:

MUCOCUTANEOUS FEATURES

- Pyoderma gangrenosum. The pathological basis of lesions of pyoderma gangrenosum is probably a vasculitis. The lesions may be single or multiple. They initially resemble boils, which subsequently break down to form necrotic ulcers with undermined purple edges (Fig. 19.5). Pyoderma gangrenosum may also occur in association with rheumatoid arthritis, multiple myeloma and leukaemia. The treatment of choice is systemic steroids, but azathioprine, minocycline or clofazimine may also be effective
- Erythema nodosum
- Perianal and buccal mucosal lesions. In Crohn's disease, anal examination may reveal fleshy tags, fissures, and perianal fistulae. The buccal mucosa may be oedematous and ulcerated, and the lips may be swollen as a result of a granulomatous cheilitis

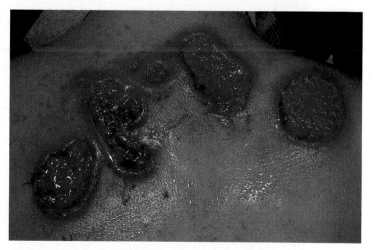

Fig. 19.5 Pyoderma gangrenosum.

HYPERLIPIDAEMIA

Both primary and secondary hyperlipidaemic states may be associated with lipid deposits in the skin, known as xanthomas. There are several different clinical types of xanthomas. Orange–yellow lipid deposits in the eyelid skin are known as xanthelasma (Fig. 19.6). Only a proportion of patients with xanthelasma have a demonstrable elevation of plasma lipids. Tuberous xanthomas occur as yellowish nodules, usually over bony prominences (Fig. 19.7). Tendinous xanthomas, as their name suggests, are deposits of lipid in association with tendons, often involving the Achilles tendons and extensor tendons on the dorsa of the hands. Deposits of lipid in the skin creases of the hands (xanthoma striatum palmare) appear to be particularly associated with primary type III hyperlipidaemia. Eruptive xanthomas are crops of yellowish papules which occur in association with marked hypertriglyceridaemia.

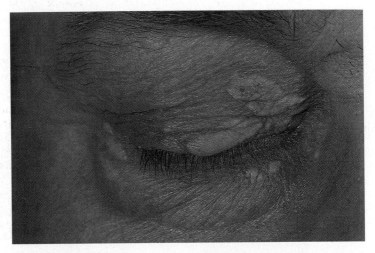

Fig. 19.6 Xanthelasma.

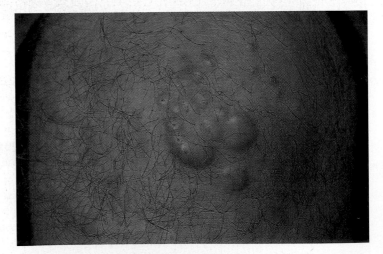

Fig. 19.7 Tuberous xanthomas.

AMYLOIDOSIS

In systemic amyloidosis, amyloid deposits in the tongue produce macroglossia, and cutaneous deposits are visible as yellowish, waxy, purpuric plaques around the eyes and in the perianal area.

SARCOIDOSIS

Sarcoidosis is a multisystem granulomatous disorder of unknown aetiology. There are a number of patterns of skin involvement in sarcoidosis, including the following.

SKIN PATTERNS

- Erythema nodosum. These tender, erythematous nodules on the legs are the result of a panniculitis (see Chapter 16). One of the commonest presentations of sarcoidosis is the erythema nodosum—arthropathy—bilateral hilar lymphadenopathy syndrome
- Lupus pernio. The skin of the nose and ears is involved in the granulomatous process, and becomes swollen and purplish in colour
- Scar sarcoid. Sarcoid granulomata localize in old scar tissue, making the scars prominent
- Papules, nodules and plaques. These often have an orange—brown colour. Plaques may be psoriasiform in appearance

LIVER DISEASE AND THE SKIN

Changes in the skin and nails which occur in association with chronic liver disease include the following:

SKIN AND NAIL CHANGES

- Palmar erythema
- Pruritus: in cholestatic liver disease
- Spider naevi: in a superior vena caval distribution
- Xanthelasma: in primary biliary cirrhosis
- White nails (Terry's nails)
- Pigmentary changes: in addition to jaundice, patients with long-standing cholestatic liver disease may also have marked melanin pigmentation. Patients suffering from haemochromatosis have generalized bronze—brown hyperpigmentation which is produced by a combination of iron and melanin

CUTANEOUS MANIFESTATIONS OF SYSTEMIC MALIGNANCY

Cutaneous metastases

Malignant tumours may metastasize to the skin, and tumours of renal, ovarian, gastrointestinal, breast and bronchial origin are those most likely to do so (Fig. 19.8). Cutaneous metastases usually present as pink nodules, and occur most frequently on the scalp and anterior trunk. Scalp metastases may produce areas of alopecia (alopecia neoplastica).

Lymphatic extension of carcinoma to the skin may produce an area of inflammatory induration resembling cellulitis known as 'carcinoma erysipelatoides'.

Metastasis of ovarian or gastrointestinal carcinoma via the ligamentum teres can present as an umbilical nodule (Sister Joseph's nodule).

Miscellaneous cutaneous signs of underlying malignancy

1 *Dermatomyositis* (see Chapter 17).
2 *Acanthosis nigricans.* This is a warty, hyperpigmented thickening of skin in the flexures (Fig. 19.9). The palms of the hands may also be affected, producing an appearance known as 'tripe palms'. The commonest associated malignancy is an adenocarcinoma of the gastrointestinal tract. However,

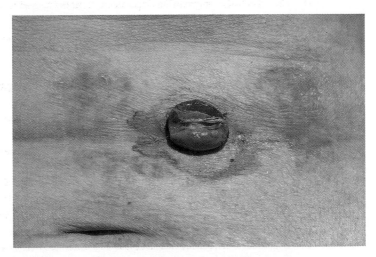

Fig. 19.8 Cutaneous metastasis from carcinoma of the oesophagus.

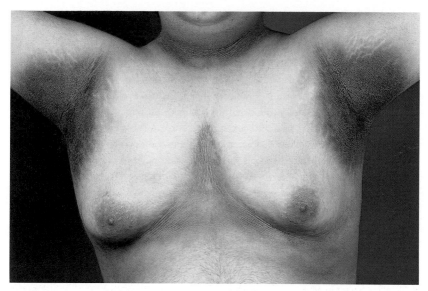

Fig. 19.9 Acanthosis nigricans.

'malignant' acanthosis nigricans is relatively rare, whereas flexural acanthosis nigricans is extremely common in the obese and is unrelated to systemic problems.

3 *Generalized pruritus.* Generalized itching may be associated with a wide variety of systemic malignancies.

4 *Thrombophlebitis migrans.* This is particularly associated with carcinoma of the pancreas.

5 *Acquired ichthyosis.* Ichthyosis developing for the first time in adult life may be associated with a lymphoma.

6 *Bullous pemphigoid* (see Chapter 14).

7 *Erythema multiforme.* An erythema multiforme-like eruption may accompany systemic neoplasia.

8 *The sign of Leser Trélat.* This is the sudden development of a profusion of seborrhoeic warts, as a manifestation of systemic malignancy.

9 *Bullous pyoderma gangrenosum.* This may occur with leukaemia and myeloma.

10 *Acquired hypertrichosis lanuginosa.* The sudden growth of profuse vellus hair over the face and body is a rare sign of underlying neoplastic disease.

11 *Necrolytic migratory erythema.* This is a distinctive eruption associated with a pancreatic glucagonoma.

12 *Flushing* and a rosacea-like eruption are cutaneous features of the carcinoid syndrome.

13 *Erythema gyratum repens.* This rare skin marker of malignancy is a bizarre patterned erythema resembling 'wood grain'.

LEUKAEMIA AND THE SKIN

There are numerous cutaneous changes which may accompany leukaemia, or be provoked by the drugs used in its treatment.

Common presenting features of acute leukaemia include purpura, bruising, and bleeding from the gums, and the skin may be directly involved in the form of leukaemic infiltrates. Disseminated herpes zoster (herpes zoster with numerous outlying vesicles) may accompany leukaemia, as may a severe bullous form of pyoderma gangrenosum, and Sweet's disease (acute febrile neutrophilic dermatosis).

BONE MARROW TRANSPLANTATION

Graft-versus-host disease (GVHD) following bone marrow transplantation affects the skin, liver and gut. The earliest sign of GVHD in the skin, which usually occurs within 2–3 weeks of the transplant, is a morbilliform (measles-like) eruption accompanied by erythema of the hands and feet. Occasionally these changes progress to toxic epidermal necrolysis (see Chapter 14). In chronic GVHD changes occur in the skin and buccal mucosa which are clinically identical to those seen in lichen planus (see Chapter 15). A later manifestation of chronic GVHD is the development of scleroderma-like changes (see Chapter 17).

PURPURA

Purpura is produced by extravasation of red cells into the skin, and has numerous causes. The lesions do not blanch on pressure.

Causes of purpura include vasculitis (see Chapter 16), quantitative or qualitative platelet abnormalities, drugs (e.g. carbromal), amyloidosis, dysproteinaemias, and infections (e.g. meningococcaemia).

AIDS AND THE SKIN

Patients suffering from the acquired immunodeficiency syndrome (AIDS) are at increased risk of developing a number of mucocutaneous problems.

1 Oral candidiasis and *Candida* intertrigo.

2 Oral 'hairy leukoplakia': clinically this presents as ribbed white areas along the sides of the tongue. Evidence suggests that human papillomaviruses and viruses of the herpes group are involved in producing hairy leukoplakia.

3 Gingivitis.

4 Seborrhoeic dermatitis: this is often severe, and is probably related to proliferation of, or an altered response to, *Pityrosporum* yeasts.

5 Itchy folliculitis: the aetiology of this non-specific pruritic folliculitis is unknown.

6 Staphylococcal infection, shingles, molluscum contagiosum, and dermatophyte fungal infection occur more commonly in AIDS patients.

7 Episodes of herpes simplex are more frequent and more severe.

8 Perianal warts tend to be more florid and more difficult to treat.

9 Kaposi's sarcoma: a tumour which is thought to arise from vascular endothelium. Lesions are usually multiple, and may affect any part of the skin, as well as internal organs. Kaposi's sarcoma is rarely the cause of death in AIDS patients, who usually succumb to intercurrent infection. It is a radiosensitive tumour.

Skin and the Psyche

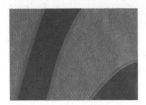

If you happen to have a wart on your nose or forehead, you cannot help imagining that no one in the world has anything else to do but stare at your wart, laugh at it, and condemn you for it, even though you have discovered America. (Fyodor Dostoevsky, *The Idiot*)

Patients with skin disease often ask 'Is it caused by nerves doctor?'. 'Nerves' is a sort of generic term in this context, but the patient is usually trying to establish if they can attribute their skin problem to a stressful situation. In fact, very few skin disorders are directly related to psychological disturbance, although sometimes 'nerves' seems much simpler than four words of inexplicable Latin mumbo jumbo. There is certainly some evidence that psoriasis and atopic eczema may be exacerbated by stress, but the pathomechanics of such an association are obscure. Other conditions in which emotional stress has been claimed to play a part in some cases include alopecia areata and acute pompholyx.

There is no doubt, however, that skin disease has psychological effects on the patient, and can significantly affect the quality of their life. Skin disease is visible to others, it carries the taint of contagion, and it is something which is socially unacceptable because of public ignorance and superstition. It requires considerable courage for an individual with a chronic dermatosis of the face or hands to work in an occupation which involves contact with the public. They will be aware that their skin is being scrutinized and that any form of physical contact, such as shaking hands or collecting change, provokes apprehension. In certain ethnic groups where marriages are arranged, the presence of skin disease may compromise marriage prospects, and cause considerable emotional distress. Infections with ectoparasites sometimes have marked psychological effects. Patients feel unclean, and these feelings can persist long after the problem has been eradicated.

There are some skin disorders which are directly related to psychological problems, and these include the following:

DERMATITIS ARTEFACTA

This is the dermatological equivalent of the Munchausen syndrome. Patients with dermatitis artefacta produce their skin lesions to satisfy a psychological need, but what benefit they derive from their actions is usually not obvious. They will vehemently deny that the lesions are self-induced if challenged. As a group they are distinct from malingerers, who consciously imitate or produce an illness for a deliberate end.

Artefactual skin lesions may be produced in a number of different ways including rubbing, scratching, picking, gouging, puncturing, cutting, sucking, biting, the application of heat or caustics, or the injection of milk, blood, and faecal material (Fig. 20.1). Limb oedema may be simulated by the intermittent application of a tourniquet. Lesions tend to have bizarre geometric shapes which do not conform to natural disease—no dermatosis has square, rectangular or triangular lesions. Often the lesions are more numerous on the side of the body opposite the dominant hand. If a caustic material has been used to induce lesions this may trickle off the main area of damage to produce tell-tale streaks at the margins. Even when suspected artefactual lesions are covered by occlusive dressings, patients will often manage to insert knitting needles under the dressings,

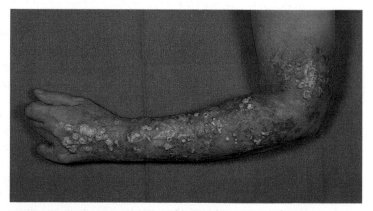

Fig. 20.1 Dermatitis artefacta—in this case probably the result of inoculation of faeces into the skin.

or push sharp instruments through them, in order to continue damaging the skin.

Dermatitis artefacta is commoner in women, most of whom are adolescents or young adults. Many have some connection with the health professions, either directly or via family members. The history is devoid of any useful information about the evolution of their lesions. The impression conveyed is that one minute the skin was normal, and the next it was blemished. This 'hollow history' is characteristic, as is a striking complacency about what are often extremely disfiguring lesions ('*la belle indifference*'). One patient we have seen, who had extensive suppuration of the left arm, probably produced by the inoculation of faeces, said 'Yes, it is rather unpleasant isn't it, I wonder if you could arrange for someone to take it off'.

The psychopathology of patients who produce artefacts is not uniform. Some produce lesions to draw attention to other problems, or as part of a personality disorder. In others, dermatitis artefacta represents a hysterical conversion or other hysterical reaction.

It requires considerable expertise to be able to make a confident diagnosis of dermatitis artefacta, but even experienced dermatologists see cases in which they suspect the lesions are self-induced, but they cannot be certain.

Treatment is difficult, if not impossible. Confronting the patient with the diagnosis usually produces a categorical denial, and subsequent failure to attend for follow-up. Strict occlusion of the traumatized area may allow healing, but the lesions will reappear as soon as occlusive dressings are removed. An alarming result of occlusion may be the appearance of lesions elsewhere, or the development of other symptoms, as if to compensate for inability to reach the usual sites. Psychiatric referral is often unhelpful, and many patients will refuse assistance from a psychiatrist. With most patients the situation remains at stalemate. The dermatologist does not confront them with the diagnosis, and they continue to visit the dermatologist. It is probably a 'you know that I know that you know' situation, but as long as suspicions are not voiced it seems to suit the patients' needs, and they are quite happy to continue attending for follow-up.

The course of this disorder is often protracted. Recovery usually has nothing to do with successful medical treatment, but occurs because of increasing maturity, marriage, or having a family.

DERMATOLOGICAL PATHOMIMICRY

Dermatological pathomimicry is distinct from dermatitis artefacta. Patients with this syndrome either deliberately perpetuate their skin disease, or reproduce a pre-existing skin disorder. Having been appraised of the aetiology of their skin disease, they use this knowledge to reproduce the lesions when under emotional stress, to obtain sympathy, or in an effort to avoid an unpleasant situation with which they cannot cope. Examples of the type of illness used by patients for pathomimicry include allergic contact dermatitis, drug reactions, and chronic leg ulceration.

Patients usually respond to positive direct psychotherapy.

DERMATOLOGICAL NON-DISEASE (DYSMORPHOPHOBIA)

In this condition patients complain of severe symptomatology localized to certain parts of the body, most commonly the face, scalp and perineum, but without any objective evidence of disease. The complaints include dysaesthesias such as burning, itching, or throbbing pain; too much or too little hair on the face or scalp, or altered texture of scalp hair; the belief that they are the source of an offensive odour. These delusional beliefs or perceptions of abnormal sensations are a consuming preoccupation for the patient. A common presentation is a female patient complaining of a burning sensation in the perineum. She will already have seen many doctors, and will have undergone various investigations, all with negative results. The perineum looks completely normal, and *is* completely normal, but it does not *feel* completely normal to the patient.

In many cases depression is part of the picture, and affected individuals may commit suicide. Untreated, the condition will continue indefinitely, but some patients will respond to treatment with antidepressants and psychotherapy.

DELUSIONS OF PARASITOSIS (PARASITOPHOBIA)

An experienced dermatologist will recognize cases of this condition from the referral letter, and will often arrange to see the patient at the end of a clinic, because the consultation is usually extremely lengthy. The typical parasitophobic is an anxious individual, often a middle-aged or elderly woman. They often contact their local university department of zoology or museums to identify 'parasites', and will be well known to companies specializing in pest eradication, who may have visited their home to 'disinfest' the premises. Members of the family may have been barred from visiting their home because of the risk of contagion, and patients may have isolated themselves from friends and acquaintances because of their fear of passing the 'infestation' on to them. Because of their absolute conviction that they are infested they may have convinced their family, friends, and even their general practitioner of the reality of their problem (shared delusion).

Parasitophobics often describe a feeling of itching, biting or 'crawling' in the skin, and state that when this occurs they are able to remove a small 'insect' or 'worm' from a skin lesion. When asked to demonstrate typical skin lesions they will often point to Campbell de Morgan spots, senile lentigines, or other minor blemishes. Typical 'specimens' are presented to the doctor wrapped in pieces of paper or adhesive tape, and kept in a match box. These should always be examined under the microscope, because they just might contain parasites, but usually they contain fragments of cotton and skin debris.

It is impossible to persuade these patients that parasites are not responsible for their condition. If they are shown that their specimens are simple debris they remain unconvinced, and may even suggest that the parasites are so small that an electron microscope will be required to demonstrate them. In this situation the most lucid, eloquent discourse will fall upon deaf ears—the patient's beliefs remain unshaken, and the doctor retires from the conflict feeling more than somewhat jaded.

Delusions of parasitosis may occur in association with organic brain disease such as senile dementia and cerebral arteriosclerosis, but the majority of patients are said to fall into one of three diagnostic categories: paranoia, paranoid schizophrenia, or involutional depression in an individual whose pre-morbid personality was obsessive.

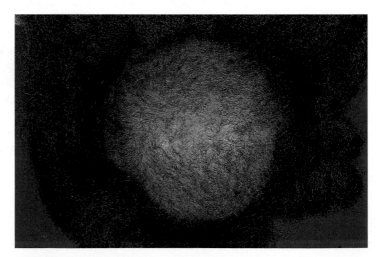

Fig. 20.2 Trichotillomania.

Effective treatment is difficult, and many parasitophobics continue with their delusions for years. Confrontation rarely achieves anything. Parasitophobics often refuse psychiatric help because they do not accept that they have a mental illness, and cannot see how a psychiatrist could help with what to them is a physical disorder. However, if possible, a psychiatrist should be involved, because expertise in treating the background psychopathology is required. The neuroleptic drug pimozide may be of benefit, if one can persuade the patients to take it.

OBSESSIVE–COMPULSIVE HABITS

Trichotillomania

Trichotillomania means compulsive plucking of hair. The scalp is involved most often, but the eyebrows and eyelashes may be affected. A mild form of trichotillomania may be observed in libraries, where engrossed students compulsively twist locks of hair around their fingers, but rarely pluck it out unless examinations are approaching! The clinical picture is of patches of hair loss containing hairs of varying length. Often the crown of the head is affected, and the hair at the margins is of normal length (Fig. 20.2). The underlying scalp is usually normal, but may be excoriated.

Trichotillomania in childhood is often transient. However, it may be a manifestation of disturbed behaviour or serious psychiatric illness, particularly in adults.

Neurotic excoriations

Neurotic excoriations are encountered much more frequently in women than in men. The lesions are produced by picking and gouging, and are usually scattered over the arms, upper trunk and face. More recent lesions are usually interspersed with scars from previous excoriations. Acne excoriée is a variant of this condition in which minimal acne lesions are repeatedly picked and gouged, leaving scars when the lesions heal.

Patients with this problem have obsessive–compulsive personalities, and picking the skin appears to provide relief of unconscious aggression and tension.

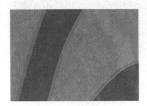

Cutaneous Drug Reactions

There are only two types of drug — those that don't work and those that have side-effects. (Bruno Handel FRCS)

INTRODUCTION

The skin is one of the commonest sites for unwanted drug effects (a better term than 'side-effects'), although estimates of the frequency of such reactions vary considerably. Drug reactions are probably under-reported and often go unrecognized.

There is also no doubt that skin disorders wholly unrelated to drug ingestion are labelled erroneously. It is important not to jump to conclusions: we have seen herpes simplex, seborrhoeic dermatitis, acne, scabies, pityriasis rosea, pityriasis versicolor and chickenpox all labelled as drug reactions. There are many people who state they are 'allergic to penicillin', but who are not.

Unfortunately there are no reliable *in vitro* tests for establishing that a rash is due to a drug. Simple *in vivo* tests, such as prick testing and patch testing, have a limited place in specific situations, but usually yield no useful information.

Cutaneous drug reactions may be due to several different mechanisms.

CAUSES OF DRUG REACTIONS

- Simple intolerance
- Hypersensitivity reactions of Types I, II, III and IV
- Pharmacokinetic disturbances
- Drug interactions
- Complex interactions between host, drug and environment (e.g. light)

Note, however, that even if the mechanism(s) for a particular reaction is known (and it often isn't), a test may not be appropriate because the reaction is not to the drug itself, but to a drug-complex or metabolite which occurs only *in vivo* after ingestion.

The only definitive test is direct challenge with the suspected agent, but this may be impossible or unethical in many circumstances. For these reasons, proving that a specific eruption was due to a specific drug is difficult, and judgements usually have to be made on clinical grounds alone.

DRUG REACTION PATTERNS

However, all is not lost! Some drugs are much more prone to induce cutaneous drug reaction patterns than others. Drugs which commonly provoke skin reactions are as follows:

DRUGS CAUSING SKIN REACTIONS

- Antibiotics (especially penicillin, semi-synthetic penicillins and sulphonamides)
- Non-steroidal anti-inflammatory drugs
- Hypnotics
- Tranquillizers

Furthermore, there are a number of well-defined clinical drug reaction patterns.

COMMON CUTANEOUS DRUG REACTION PATTERNS

- Exanthematic eruptions
- Urticaria and anaphylaxis
- Exfoliative dermatitis
- Vasculitis

Continued on p. 272

COMMON CUTANEOUS DRUG REACTION PATTERNS *(Continued)*

- Fixed drug eruptions
- Lichen planus-like eruptions
- Erythema multiforme
- Acneiform eruptions
- Hair abnormalities
- Pigmentary changes
- Bullous reactions
- Photosensitivity
- Lupus erythematosus-like syndrome
- Exacerbation of pre-existing skin disease

Some of these patterns are more drug-specific, and therefore recognition of them as drug reactions may help to identify the culprit.

Exanthematic eruptions

The commonest cutaneous drug reactions are usually itchy, widespread, symmetrical, erythematous and maculopapular (Fig. 21.1): there is often a strong resemblance to a viral exanthem. The time relationship is variable: in most instances the rash begins within a few days of starting the drug, but it may begin almost immediately, or be delayed for a few weeks. Exanthematic eruptions usually fade a week or so after stopping the drug, but exfoliative dermatitis may develop if it is not withdrawn (see below and Chapter 15).

Common causes: non-steroidal anti-inflammatory drugs and antibiotics, particularly ampicillin, other semi-synthetic penicillins, sulphonamides and gentamicin.

Rarer causes: gold, barbiturates and phenothiazines.

Urticaria and anaphylaxis (see also Chapter 15)

Drug-induced urticaria may be due to a direct pharmacological action on mast cells, or to a Type I or Type III hypersensitivity reaction.

Occasionally, drugs may trigger a major anaphylactic reaction, with or without urticaria, which can be fatal unless treated very rapidly. Unfortunately, there is no known way of predicting this disaster.

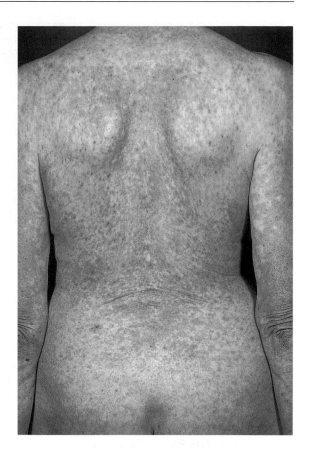

Fig. 21.1 A typical exanthematic eruption due to an antibiotic.

Common causes: aspirin, opiates (direct), penicillins, cephalosporins, pollen vaccines and toxoids (immune).

Eczema

Type IV hypersensitivity reactions to topical medicaments are common, and give rise to a contact dermatitis (see Chapter 7). Figure 21.2 shows a woman who was given eye drops containing an aminoglycoside antibiotic. Occasionally, a topically sensitized patient may receive the compound (or a closely related chemical) systemically. The result is a severe, widespread, eczematous reaction.

Common causes: lanolin in creams and bandages; preservatives (parabens, ethylenediamine) in creams; topical anaesthetics (*not* lignocaine);

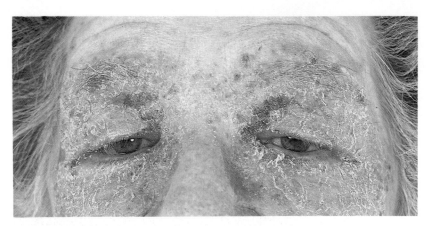

Fig. 21.2 Contact sensitivity to neomycin.

topical antihistamines; topical antibiotics, especially aminoglycosides, in creams and drops.

Exfoliative dermatitis

Drugs are one of the four important causes of exfoliative dermatitis (see Chapter 15).

Common causes: prominent offenders are sulphonamides and sulphonylureas, gold, phenytoin, allopurinol and barbiturates.

Vasculitis (see Chapter 16)

Drug ingestion is a common trigger for vasculitis.

Common causes: in our experience, thiazides are the drugs most frequently implicated, but vasculitis has also been reported with captopril, cimetidine, quinidine, sulphonamides and some others.

Fixed drug eruptions

Fixed drug eruptions are one of the most curious events encountered in dermatological practice. The reaction occurs in the same place(s) every time the offending drug is taken. They are often misdiagnosed as recurrent eczema or ringworm.

A round or oval patch of dusky erythema develops, often with a purplish centre (Fig. 21.3), and sometimes a central bulla. This fades to leave

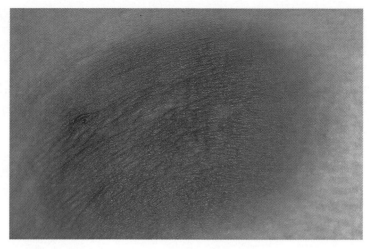

Fig. 21.3 Fixed drug reaction to a sulphonamide.

post-inflammatory hyperpigmentation. There may be only one lesion, or the reaction may occur at multiple sites. Fixed eruptions can occur anywhere, but the limbs and genitalia are favoured sites.

Common causes: laxatives containing phenolphthalein, sulphonamides, dapsone, tetracyclines, barbiturates and chlordiazepoxide.

Lichen planus-like eruptions

Lichen planus-like (sometimes known as 'lichenoid') reactions are rare, but can be severe. The eruption is occasionally indistinguishable from idiopathic lichen planus, but more commonly there is an eczematous element, and there is much more scaling. In severe cases an exfoliative dermatitis may develop (see above and Chapter 15).

Causes: antimalarial drugs; some beta-blockers; sulphonylureas; gold. Thiazides may cause lichen planus-like eruptions on light-exposed surfaces.

Erythema multiforme (see Chapter 15)

So many things seem to be able to trigger erythema multiforme that it is usually difficult to be certain whether a drug is responsible.

Suggested drug causes: barbiturates; long-acting sulphonamides; co-trimoxazole; rifampicin.

Acneiform eruptions

Skin changes resembling acne vulgaris occur with several drugs. The changes tend to be monomorphic, consisting largely of papulopustules. There are seldom comedones present.

Causes: corticosteroids (both topical and systemic), adrenocorti-cotrophic hormone (ACTH), androgenic drugs, lithium and iodides. Some drugs also exacerbate pre-existing acne (see below).

Hair abnormalities

As discussed in Chapter 13, drugs may be responsible for hair loss or excessive hair growth.

Pigmentary changes

Several drugs cause pigmentary changes (Table 21.1).

Heavy metals such as silver may be deposited in the skin following industrial exposure or ingestion (e.g. in anti-smoking lozenges).

DRUG-INDUCED PIGMENTARY CHANGES

Colour	Drug
Characteristic generalized reddish-brown hue	Clofazimine (used in leprosy)
Yellow	Mepacrine Carotene
Blue–black	Chloroquine (especially on shins) Minocycline (in high dosage) Amiodarone (on light-exposed sites)
Purplish	Chlorpromazine
Brown	Oestrogens (= chloasma)

Table 21.1 Drugs causing cutaneous pigmentary changes.

Bullous reactions

There are several ways in which drugs may induce blistering.

DRUG-INDUCED BLISTERING

- In fixed drug eruptions
- Drugs may induce pemphigus and pemphigoid (see Chapter 14)
- Drugs may exacerbate porphyria cutanea tarda
- Nalidixic acid may cause a dramatic phototoxic bullous reaction
- Barbiturates may cause bullae on pressure points, usually in patients unconscious due to overdose

Photosensitivity

There are three main types of reaction.

PHOTOSENSITIVE REACTIONS

- Exacerbation of underlying disease
- Direct phototoxic reaction
- Photoallergic reaction

In phototoxic reactions, the dose of the drug and the intensity of ultraviolet exposure may both be important: if critical levels are not reached the reaction may not develop. This can be confusing if the drug has been taken on a number of occasions.

Patients complain that exposure to the sun causes a burning sensation followed by erythema, swelling and, later, eczematous changes on lightexposed areas (Fig. 21.4).

Common causes: phenothiazines; sulphonamides; tetracyclines; thiazides. Demethylchlortetracycline can cause photo-onycholysis. Bullae due to nalidixic acid have been mentioned above.

Lupus erythematosus-like syndrome

A rare but important drug reaction is the induction of a syndrome closely resembling systemic lupus erythematosus.

Causes: many agents have been incriminated, including hydralazine, isoniazid, penicillin, procainamide and griseofulvin.

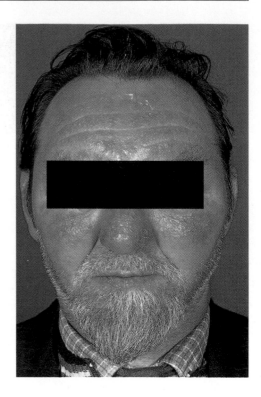

Fig. 21.4 Photosensitivity to a sulphonamide.

Exacerbation of pre-existing disease

Some drugs may produce a deterioration in certain skin disorders. Notable examples are:

1 acne—androgenic drugs (e.g. danazol, stanozolol), oral contraceptives and corticosteroids;

2 porphyrias — all clinical features, including cutaneous photosensitivity, may be worsened by drug ingestion, particularly barbiturates and oestrogens;

3 psoriasis—lithium, antimalarials;

4 systemic lupus erythematosus—penicillin and sulphonamides may produce deterioration.

CONCLUSION

If you use all the clinical information at your disposal it is often possible to come to a reasonable conclusion.

CLINICAL INFORMATION

- A good history
- A careful examination
- Elimination of other skin diseases
- Recognition of the clinical reaction pattern
- Matching the reaction with the most likely offender *and*
- Tests, where appropriate (possibly including a challenge)

CHAPTER 22

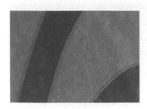

Treatment of
Skin Disease

If it's dry, wet it. If it's wet, dry it. Congratulations, you are now a dermatologist!
(Anonymous)

The above witticism is oft-quoted by non-dermatologists as an assessment of the scope of dermatological therapeutics. An alternative calumny relates to a dermatologist murmuring an unintelligible Latin name as a diagnosis, and then always prescribing a topical steroid. Both these quips are far from the truth, as dermatologists have an extensive therapeutic armamentarium at their disposal. In the past, it must be admitted, many of the available topical therapies were cosmetically unacceptable and often malodorous—if the skin disease did not render the patient a social pariah, the treatment could be relied upon to do so. However, in recent years, most topical therapies are not only more effective, but also cosmetically much more acceptable.

This chapter is designed to provide an overview of the principles of topical therapy.

An ideal topical preparation for the management of skin disease would penetrate well, but remain entirely localized within the skin, thus avoiding potential problems from systemic effects. In practice this is difficult to achieve, and any agent which penetrates the stratum corneum is absorbed to some extent.

Topical preparations consist of an active ingredient (or ingredients) and a material in which this is suspended—a base. These must be compatible. The stratum corneum forms a barrier to penetration of externally applied agents, and the activity of any topically applied drug is determined by its ability to transgress this barrier. Hydration of the stratum corneum impairs its barrier function, and this can be achieved by occlusion of the skin. Penetration of a topical steroid may be considerably enhanced by occluding an area of skin with polythene. However, if large areas of skin are occluded the amount of steroid absorbed will be sufficient to produce significant systemic effects. Bases containing urea also hydrate the stratum corneum and enhance penetration of their active ingredients. Dimethyl sulphoxide (DMSO) is a solvent which penetrates skin extremely rapidly, and is used as a vehicle for the antiviral agent idoxuridine.

BASES

Bases include creams, oily creams, ointments, lotions, gels, and pastes. A cream is an oil-in-water emulsion which is relatively non-greasy and has only limited emollient activity. Creams are cosmetically acceptable and can be used to treat either moist or dry skin conditions. Oily creams are water-in-oil emulsions which combine good emollient properties with cosmetic acceptability and are therefore of benefit in dry skin conditions. Ointments are greasy preparations which have emollient and occlusive properties. The occlusive effect of an ointment results in hydration of the stratum corneum and enhanced penetration of the active ingredient of the ointment. The benefits of ointments are offset by a lack of cosmetic acceptability. Ointments are messy and stick to clothing. If used on the hands they transfer to everything touched—an obvious disadvantage to someone employed in clerical work. Lotions are fluid preparations which have a cooling effect due to evaporation. They are useful in the management of moist, exudative skin lesions, and also in dermatoses affecting the scalp. Clear, non-greasy gels are designed for use on hairy parts of the body, where they are cosmetically acceptable. Pastes are powders, usually mixed with soft paraffin, and are protective—for example, in the prevention of maceration of the skin around a discharging ulcer.

The choice of a particular base should be determined by the type of skin problem and the sites affected. It is, for example, wholly inappropriate to prescribe a steroid ointment for daytime use on the scalp, because it is too messy. A gel or lotion preparation should be used instead. Similarly, a lotion is not the correct base for ichthyotic skin, where an oily cream or ointment are more appropriate.

Bases are mixtures of several components, formulated to provide stability and freedom from microbial contamination. Random dilution of a topical preparation will dilute the preservatives in the base and significantly shorten its shelf-life.

COMMUNICATION AND PATIENT COMPLIANCE

Topical therapy demands a great deal of the patient, and the effort required by the patient ought to be matched by the provision of precise instructions by the doctor. Verbal instructions are not sufficient if multiple topical therapies are prescribed. For example, a patient suffering from psoriasis might be given a tar shampoo, a scalp lotion, a mild topical steroid cream to use in the flexures, and a dithranol preparation for short contact therapy to plaques on the trunk and limbs. If the patient has only recently developed psoriasis, and is not familiar with its treatment, the provision of multiple therapies without clear instructions could easily lead to confusion.

Do not expect patients who depart for work at the crack of dawn to adhere strictly to instructions to wash their hair every morning and use a topical medication twice daily. Modify the treatment schedule to suit the individual. If you are prescribing a preparation which is messy to use and/or malodorous, warn the patient about this. For example, dithranol stains, and benzoyl peroxide bleaches, and lack of prior warning could lead to ruined clothing and bed-sheets.

QUANTITIES PRESCRIBED

It is important when prescribing topical therapy to consider the area to be covered and the frequency of application before assessing the quantity of a topical agent required by the patient. For example, there is little point in prescribing a 30 g tube of an emollient to be used over the entire body surface after bathing—a repeat prescription would be required after one application, because this is the approximate amount required for a single application over the whole body surface of an adult. Topical therapies are available in a variety of container sizes. You will need to check the available sizes before prescribing, as they vary from product to product. Topical steroids, for example, may be marketed in 5, 15, 25, 30, 50 or 100 g tubes, depending on the manufacturer. Most emollients are available in 50 and 100 g tubes and 500 g tubs or dispensers.

Underprescribing and overprescribing are both common. One does not require 100 g of cream to treat a small patch of eczema on the leg— most of the tube will languish in a drawer or bathroom cabinet until its shelf-life is long expired, or may be inappropriately used by another member of the family. Overprescribing of potent topical steroids may encourage the use of excessive amounts, with the risk of local and systemic adverse effects.

TOPICAL STEROIDS

There are a number of topical steroids, and they may be divided into several groups according to potency. Hydrocortisone preparations are the weakest. A few hydrocortisone preparations are more potent because their bases contain urea, and this enhances penetration of the stratum corneum. Modification of the basic steroid skeleton by fluorination or esterification produces steroids of much greater potency (Table 22.1).

Choice of preparation

The most appropriate topical steroid for a given situation should be determined by the type and severity of the condition being treated, the sites affected, and the age of the patient. The skin disorders which are steroid responsive have been delineated in previous chapters, and include various types of eczema, lichen planus, psoriasis of the scalp, flexures, hands and feet, and discoid lupus erythematosus. Topical steroids must not be used in the treatment of viral, bacterial or fungal infections of the skin. In general, a severe dermatosis should be treated with a potent steroid, and a mild condition with a weak steroid. In the case of a chronic dermatosis subject to periodic exacerbations a mild to moderate potency steroid can be used when the condition is quiescent, and a potent preparation to control the exacerbations.

There are regional variations in the absorption of topical steroids

STEROID POTENCY

Group	Potency	Examples
IV	Mild	1% Hydrocortisone
III	Moderately potent	Clobetasone butyrate (Eumovate) Flurandrenolone (Haelan) Hydrocortisone with urea (Alphaderm)
II	Potent	Betamethasone valerate (Betnovate) Fluocinolone acetonide (Synalar) Fluocinonide (Metosyn) Hydrocortisone butyrate (Locoid)
I	Very potent	Clobetasol propionate (Dermovate) Diflucortolone valerate (Nerisone Forte)

Table 22.1 Topical steroid potency (British National Formulary).

through the skin and their potential for local adverse effects. These variations are determined by the thickness of the stratum corneum, occlusion, for example in the flexures, and the vascularity of the area. Most facial dermatoses should only be treated with mild topical steroids, although a few conditions such as discoid lupus erythematosus will require potent preparations. Skin disease affecting the axillae, groins and sub-mammary areas should also be treated with mild topical steroids. Conversely, dermatoses of the palms and soles, where the stratum corneum is extremely thick, require potent steroids.

There is a greater risk of adverse systemic effects from the use of topical steroids in children because of the high ratio of skin surface area to body volume, particularly in infants. For this reason mild topical steroids should be used in small children. The skin of the elderly is thin, and potent steroids will exacerbate this change — their prolonged use in the elderly should therefore be avoided.

Side-effects

Side-effects are rarely seen following the use of mild topical steroids, but they are encountered more frequently in association with potent topical steroid use. Side-effects may be divided into local, occurring at the site of application of the steroid, and systemic, resulting from percutaneous absorption.

LOCAL

Atrophy of the skin. Topical steroids produce dose-related thinning of the dermis. This effect is particularly noticeable in areas where the skin is naturally relatively thin, such as the axillae, medial aspect of the upper arm, groins, and the medial aspect of the thigh. Prominent striae may develop in these areas (Fig. 22.1). On the face, cutaneous thinning and telangiectasia produce prominent erythema.

Peri-oral dermatitis. Peri-oral dermatitis is a condition usually seen in young women who have used potent topical steroids on the face for lengthy periods of time—often inappropriately for mild acne on the chin. The eruption consists of small papules and pustules on an erythematous background (Fig. 22.2) The history is virtually identical in all cases. Initially the condition appears to improve, probably because the vasoconstrictor activity of the steroid reduces erythema, and inflammatory papules become less noticeable. However, stopping treatment results in a rebound flare of the erythema, and the patient therefore considers the treatment is keeping the condition controlled and continues to apply the steroid; she may even increase the frequency of application. Eventually, as

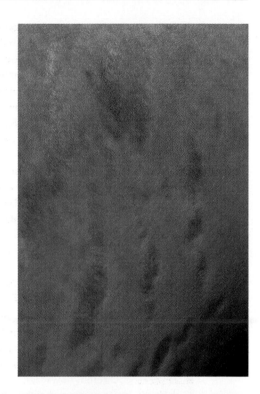

Fig. 22.1 Prominent striae on the thigh.

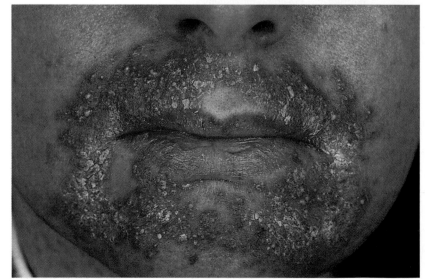

Fig 22.2 Peri-oral dermatitis.

the eruption around her mouth becomes more noticeable, she asks her doctor for something 'stronger', and is often given a more potent topical steroid.

Treatment consists of stopping the potent steroid, warning the patient about the rebound flare of erythema, and prescribing a mild topical steroid for 2–3 weeks to reduce its severity. In addition, oxytetracycline should be given in a dose of 500 mg bd, gradually reducing over a period of several weeks as the condition improves. The reason for its efficacy is unknown.

Steroid rosacea. Topical steroids will worsen pre-existing rosacea, and can precipitate a rosacea-like eruption.

Infection. Folliculitis may occur in areas treated with topical steroids, particularly when ointments or polythene occlusion are used, and the use of steroids on moist, warm flexural areas may encourage superinfection with *Candida*. Inappropriate use of topical steroids on dermatophyte fungal infections alters the appearance of the eruption, producing so-called 'tinea incognito' (see Chapter 4). Scabies treated with topical steroids becomes extremely florid, with many burrows and a very numerous mite population (see Chapter 5).

SYSTEMIC EFFECTS

Topical steroids are absorbed through the skin, and excessive use of potent steroids may result in iatrogenic Cushing's syndrome. This problem is rarely encountered nowadays, because those prescribing potent steroids have become more familiar with their potential adverse effects, and restrict the amounts prescribed.

Children are more susceptible than adults to the systemic effects of topical steroids, and growth retardation is an important consequence of the long-term use of potent topical steroid therapy.

Index